Vitality

Quest for a healthy diet
in the wake of the low carb craze

Allison Tannis, BSc, MSc

Printed in Canada

FIN 01 17 06

Library and Archives Canada Cataloguing in Publication

Tannis, Allison
    Vitality : quest for a healthy diet in the way of the low carb craze / Allison Tannis.

ISBN 0-9737821-0-2

    1. Nutrition. I. Title.

RA784.T35 2005   613.2   C2005-902436-4

Table of Contents

Quest for a healthy diet
in the wake of the low-carb craze

By Allison Tannis, BSc, MSc

Forward:

At no time in my life have I felt so passionate and sympathetic to the North American society. We are utterly confused about what to eat. People are frustrated with the way they look and with the lack of clear information to help them understand the mystery of food and diets. For this reason, I have written this book - a clear and scientifically supported account of the major issues facing our carbohydrate-confused society. I truly believe that with knowledge each of us can hold the power to live healthier lives. With all that we know as scientists it is ridiculous to have people suffering from obesity and malnutrition in a society where there is no shortage of good food. If this book helps one person learn one way that they can make better food choices to live better, than it has been a success.

My love for the world we live in, and my belief that we all have the right to be healthy, are not my only motivation driving me to write this book. We have all lost a close loved one to disease. Some of us have lost loved ones to diseases that could have been prevented with a good diet.

1

About one-third of deaths from disease could be prevented through dietary means. I have watched the lack of a good diet take away one of my most loved family members. If only he had understood the basics of diet and its effects on his health; if only someone had take the time to explain it in an easy to understand way, he may have lived a long healthy life. Instead, his passing has opened my eyes to the need for better prevention. Our health care systems are designed to fix the ill – not to prevent getting ill. This may be our Achilles' heal. Education can save lives.

Arm yourself with the facts. Learn the science of nutrition – it is much easier than you think. And, with the knowledge of nutrition, you can make choices to give your body the items it needs to function properly.

If I could make one wish, it would be for everyone to enjoy the wonderful feeling of wellness when they eat right and take care of themselves. You will have more energy, the world will look brighter and all your aches and pains will seem farther away. Why not try it? Give healthy eating a chance. You'll appreciate it. If you truly try the results may save your life.

I hope you all enjoy this book and its messages. I hope that it offers some help to many of you who are confused about fat, carbohydrates (carbs), protein, and more. However, as you read this book please remember that you cannot change who you are, how you eat or what you look like over night. It will take time. It took me 4 years to totally convert my diet and dietary patterns from a typical healthy North American diet, to the perfect diet (with a few cheats of course.) Smile! You're on your way to healthy living. Sit back, put your feet up and read your way to health. Its time to let North American's understand healthy eating. Enjoy!

Acknowledgements:

There are so many people who have supported me and encouraged me along the way. Many fueled my curiosity for science: at home the patience for my messy experiments; at school the extra work when I asked, the encouragement to enter science fairs; at secondary school my biology teacher teaching that science need not be complicated and can be taught to anyone if the right analogies are used; at university my graduate supervisor believed in me to use my abilities to translate science into everyday terms and share it with others; and professionally my first boss believed in me and gave me the opportunity to reach for the stars. For this, I thank all of you. The world of science is so fascinating that I awake each morning optimistic and curious as to what interesting fact I might learn that day. Each time I start up my computer and smile with wonder as to what new study has been published to answer our questions about the world or to cause us to ask new questions.

And, to my husband — my biggest fan, I could not have done this without you.

Because each of you believed in me, I do what I do today. Thank you. You made it possible – thanks.

Introduction:

Why is it that we are obsessed with weight loss? Is it because we are truly an obese society or because we are fixated with the way we look? Images on magazines at the check-out aisle, commercials, movies, and advertisements are full of young, perfect, thin people. Runways are filled with starving models. Is it our desire to be thin, to look like these media images that drive us to flip-flop from diet to diet? Just think about the diets that have come and gone over the last few decades. In the 1960s, the Drinking Man's diet proclaimed that alcohol would help with weight loss or the famous specific food diets such as the Cabbage Soup Diet, the Water Diet, the Rice Diet and the Grapefruit Diet. Not to mention the Five Day Miracle, Eat Right for your Blood type and the I Love New York diets. Each diet promised quick, easy and painless weight loss. Each was announced to be a "break-through" in dietary theories. Each claimed to be the diet that would end the need for dieting. With each new diet to hit the market, we flocked to stores to buy books and products that promised to help us attain weight loss and the body image we crave. We've created an epidemic of yo-yo dieting.

Every year, 50 million Americans attempt to follow a "lose weight quick" idea and fail to adopt a permanent, healthy lifestyle. The only results of these 50 million Americans are large dollar sales for diet marketers, another round of yo-yo dieting and compromised health. In fact, scientists have discovered that women who reported intentionally losing 10 pounds or more on a diet, had a lower immunity level. Furthermore, the more frequent the intentional weight loss the worse off the person's immune system was.[1]

Therefore, yo-yo dieting is more costly than the price you'll pay for the next diet book. It is costly to your health – a priceless commodity. Yo-yo dieting can compromise your health and never really teaches you how to eat well.

Perhaps the larger problem of diet and diet plans today is that we're still waiting for that perfect diet: the diet of all diets. Despite the hundreds of diets that have passed the shelves of North America in the past half century, we're still not satisfied.

Obesity has been described by some as the biggest epidemic in North America. According to Dr. Keith Garleb[2], "By converting the extra seven billion pounds of fat American adults carry around their bodies, the population of the world could be fed for two days."

We are a fat nation. We are a frustrated, fat nation. We no longer understand what makes a good, healthy diet, and what can help us become thinner. In the 1980s we thought fat made us fat. The fat phobia from the 1980s drove us to reduce the amount of fats in our diets. Yet, despite eating less fat, we are still getting fatter.[3]

Therefore, diets high in fat do not appear to be the primary cause of obesity. Reductions in fat intake do not appear to work to reduce obesity. Thus, our frustration with fat grows, and in the twenty-first century a new fat concept began – the low-carb diet was the craze of the time.

In 2004, up to 3/4 of the population used some form of low-carbohydrate diet. A majority of the population felt that a low-carbohydrate diet was a good way to lose weight. And, over half of North American's believed that the low-carb trend would last forever[4]. Thus, the low-carb concept affected most North American's way of thinking when it came to carbohydrates, protein and fat. Many were left confused. Therefore, in our quest for a

6

healthy diet we need to uncover the truth about carbs, the truth about weight loss and what is a truly good, healthy diet, so we can all achieve healthy living.

Is the low-carb diet that one perfect diet we were waiting for? Is it a "good" diet? We'll never know unless we uncover the truth about high-protein/low-carbohydrate diets, in our search for a "good" diet.

The high-protein/low-carbohydrate diet started in the 1970s when Dr. Atkins first suggested a high protein diet for weight loss. High protein diets involved restrictions on carbohydrate intake. However, the fat phobia of the 1980s restricted the popularity of the high protein diet. But, at the turn of the century high-protein/low-carbohydrate diets were flooding North America. Atkin's South Beach, Zone and Stillman were just a few of these low-carbohydrate diets. Most popular was the Atkins diet. Dr. Atkins' fundamental theories on increasing dietary protein and limiting carbohydrate intake were supported by some scientific research. His theories have been shown to cause weight loss. However, negative side effects of this diet exist and there is also science that contradicts its effectiveness. This resulted in confusion about carbohydrates, fats, and proteins and how they should proportionately make up a healthy diet. The lack of knowledge created a society that is uninformed about proper dieting. Knowledge is power. It is the power to attain health. The results of uninformed dietary decisions can be tragic.

Perhaps we are not just uninformed, but misinformed. The scientific founding theories of Dr. Atkins' diet were altered and manifested in the media from a high protein diet into an anti-carb/no-carb message. The facts were lost. It's like the childhood game telephone, where the original message is gibberish by the time it reaches the final listener. The real message of this dietary theory has been completely distorted by the media and society. The result is many North American's practicing a diet that may be hazardous to their health because they do not truly understand food, diet and nutrition. The misconceptions of low-carbohydrate diets concerned physicians so much that a few found it necessary to create a physicians guide to low-carbohydrate diets.[5]

Such a cry of concern from medical practitioners advising the positive and negative effects of low-carbohydrate dieting and recommendations on how to advise patients is yet another indication to the severity of our confusion with dieting, healthy eating and weight management.

North America is facing the largest change in dietary perception it's seen in two decades. Not since we were invaded with the low fat diet in the 1980s have we seen a nation-wide change in food choices or a change that has affected people of every age, income and race. We're drowning in media messages about high-protein/low-carbohydrate diets, their promises of quick and easy weight loss and reports of their danger and ineffectiveness. However, there are no clear messages about what makes a "healthy" diet. The carbohydrate movement has left North Americans completely confused as to what a healthy diet is.

With an estimated 300,000 deaths in the United States associated with obesity each year[6], and the percentage of overweight Americans jumping from 55.9% to 64.5% in the last decade[7], the war on obesity is intensifying and the need for a quick fix is imperative. The search for a good, healthy diet is becoming desperate.

It is time to uncover the facts, the science, and the truth about protein, carbohydrates and fat. It is time to find a healthy diet.

Chapter 1:
Truth about Weight Loss

The word diet is commonly associated with the idea of losing weight, thus it is important to discuss weight loss. Obesity represents a major threat to health and quality of life. According to the International Obesity Task Force, 1.7 billion people worldwide were obese in 2003.[8] The United States Census Bureau estimates that the prevalence of adults in the United States, aged 20-74, who are overweight and obese, today stands at 65% and will reach 73% by 2008.

Why are we so fat? Some experts say that it's because humans have similar eating patterns to the rat – humans will eat until overfed. This is an evolutionary response to eat and store energy to be able to survive a future famine. However, when, if ever, does the local supermarket run out of food? We are not likely to see a famine in the near future in North America. Therefore, we never find a need to use all of this energy we are storing.

With each generation we appear to be storing more energy for this fictional upcoming famine. According to Professor Roland Auer, of the University of Calgary we are fat because we eat 15% more calories with each generation.[9] According to the World Health Organization we are fat because we've transitioned our food choices towards refined foods, food of animal origin, and increased fat. According to all of these experts, we are fat

9

because we may have genes that tell us to overeat, we eat more with each generation and we choose the wrong foods.

Why do we care if we are fat? Clothes come in all sizes and body fat is useful as it keeps us warm in the winter. What is the concern? Well, obesity is a concern because it is associated with disease. Excessive body fat is associated with an increased cancer risk. A study that observed 900,000 people for 16 years estimated that excess body fat may account for 14% of all cancer deaths in men and, 20% of cancer deaths in women.[10] This type of convincing research warns us of the danger of obesity.

Although obesity has strong genetic determinants, it is generally accepted that it results from an imbalance between food intake and daily physical activity. We eat too much food and exercise too little hence, we have an obesity problem. This is reflected in the health guidelines across North America which focuses on two particular lifestyle factors: increasing levels of physical activity and reducing the intakes of fat and sugars.

Most health experts agree that all long-term weight loss programs should include regular exercise,[11] but is exercise alone a means of weight loss? Research appears to indicate that when dietary programs are compared, there is more significant weight loss when caloric restriction and exercise are combined, than with just exercise alone. Without question physical activity is a vital part of weight management and a healthy lifestyle. Exercise promotes energy/fat balance while providing beneficial alterations to obesity/overweight-related health problems. However, many people are discouraged from exercise because they believe it has to include grueling spin classes, long distance running, painful weight lifting routines and army-like step aerobic classes.

There is disagreement among scientific experts as to how much exercise is needed to achieve weight loss and whether or not there is a dose-response effect.[12,13] For those of you who cringe at the idea of a weight loss plan that includes intense workouts such as the stair climber that makes you feel like you are climbing Mount Everest, or the rowing machine seems like its in the ocean during a hurricane - never fear. The *Journal of the American Medical Association* reported a study of women who were put on a calorie reduced diet and varying exercise programs for a year. They found that regardless of exercise intensity the women attained weight loss (average 13 to 20 lbs), maintained the weight loss and improved cardiovascular fitness.[14] In other words, you do not have to train for a marathon to lose weight. Any amount of exercise can help with weight management. Do what you can so that you will keep doing it. Conquering Everest and the ocean are not necessary to achieve weight loss. You simply need to get moving – any type of physical activity can help.

To maximize weight loss what type of physical activity is best? There has been a lot of research in exercise and energy expenditure. Scientists have been researching the various ways that the body finds energy to burn while doing exercise. When researchers investigated what happens in the body during various types of exercise, they found that the most enjoyable exercise is the most effective way to burn fat.[15]

For simplicity, we'll only discuss three types of exercise: high, medium and low intensity. Think of high intensity as being an intense spin or aerobic class, medium as a quick paced walk or a bike ride, and low intensity as a walk.

High intensity exercise requires a lot of energy quickly. During high intensity exercise the body uses carbohydrates as fuel. This carbohydrate mostly comes from the glycogen cells, or battery packs, in our muscles. Some fats are used as fuel in high intensity exercise. These fats are taken equally from the plasma (i.e. blood) and intramuscular (i.e. fat in the muscles). Intramuscular fat is the ideal source to use if you are trying to trim down or reduce the total size of your body. It is important to note that high intensity exercise is an important part of any physical activity schedule as it helps keep your heart strong and fit, as well as many other healthy benefits.

Medium intensity exercise appears to cause your body to burn the most fat per minute of the three possible exercise intensities discussed here. In fact, fats are used to create 90% of the energy required for medium intensity exercise. Medium intensity exercise is about 50% of VO_2 max, or about half of the top possible intensity you could do before falling over. Interestingly, the body burns up equal amounts of fat from the plasma and intramuscular for the first 60 minutes of medium intensity exercise. However, after 60 minutes the body seems to rely more on plasma fatty acids. Therefore, medium intensity exercise for up to one hour is the best way to trim down, as it burns a lot of intramuscular fat.

As for low intensity exercise, it also appears to be an effective way to burn fat. Researchers found that the maximum amount of intramuscular fat that can be used occurs between 45 minutes and 75 minutes of low intensity exercise. Intramuscular fat is the type of fat we want to get rid of. By burning intramuscular fat during exercise you will loose inches, and weight.

Therefore, research suggests that if weight loss or management is your goal than medium to low intensity exercise may be ideal. Take a long walk each day and enjoy the view, relax your mind and walk off the inches. Occasionally, pick up the pace or hop on a bike and do some medium intensity exercise for a shorter period of time. And, ideally get in come high intensity exercise each week to give your heart a workout.

Researchers have also investigated whether aerobic or anaerobic exercise is better for weight loss. They found that when exercise is done aerobically, (i.e. being on a treadmill at a steady, sustainable pace, in the presence of lots of oxygen) the body uses a combination of fat and carbohydrates. However, anaerobic exercise (i.e. running as quickly as possible on a treadmill, without sufficient oxygen to the muscles) the body uses mostly carbohydrates.[16] Thus, as fat contains more calories than carbohydrates it would be more beneficial to weight loss to burn fat instead of carbohydrates. This research supports the idea that medium to lower intensity exercise where your muscle are in the presence of oxygen promotes the body using fat as a fuel, the ideal source for weight loss exercise programs.

Being active at any level has its healthy benefits. However, you need not sweat buckets, strain with pain or, spend an hour panting through an aerobics class to loose weight. Just start with a walk. Get moving and you'll start to feel and look better.

Despite the large role that exercise plays in weight management, it will not be discussed in great detail here. However, it should be noted that physical activity is likely a key element to achieving a healthy weight and is key in the maintenance of a healthy body. More importantly, exercise and physical fitness are associated with increased energy, feelings of contentment and reduced risk of some diseases. Exercise is a part of a healthy lifestyle and should be a part of everyone's daily routines.

As weight loss involved caloric expenditure (i.e. physical activity) and food intake, the next step on our quest for a healthy diet is to understand food intake and weight loss. To do this let's look more closely at the two most popular types of weight loss diets of the last century: the low fat diet and the high-protein/low-carbohydrate diet.

a) Low-Carb Weight Loss

Not all weight loss is equal. There are many parts in our body that contribute to our overall weight: fat, muscle, water and bone. An overall loss in weight can be the loss of one or many of these parts. This is important to know and understand. This will help explain the heroic weight loss stories associated with the high-protein/low-carbohydrate diet.

Low-carb diets have many stories about losing weight. In fact, some stories include vast weight loss in a very short period of time. The extreme phase approach of the Atkin's diet allows for quick and immediate weight loss. However, is the quick weight loss of the low-carb diet good, sustainable or healthy?

According to researchers, the weight loss experienced with high-protein/low-carb diets is wrongly associated with the elimination of carbohydrates. Researchers believe that weight loss from a low-carb diet comes largely from a loss of water and muscle. When you do not have enough carbohydrates in your diet, your body begins to burn stored carbohydrates (e.g. glycogen) for energy, which releases a lot of water from your tissues. This water ends up in the blood vessels, increasing blood pressure which causes the kidneys to excrete the excess water, resulting in a net water loss from the body. And, of course, a net weight loss. Also, reduced carbohydrate intake influences the sodium water balance in the body, thereby resulting in further fluid loss and weight loss.

In addition, the high-protein/low-carb diet forces you to make drastic changes to your diet by requesting that from the first day on, you radically restrict your carbohydrate intake. When we restrict one particular item from our diet, the result is a decrease in total calorie consumption, as we may struggle to find alternatives to eat. Not to mention that there is an inherent trend to eat less when we are dieting as we are forced to pay attention to what we are eating. Therefore, the initial weight loss in high-protein/low-carb diets is also likely attributed to the caloric reduction which occurs naturally from dieting.

These initial causes of weight loss may explain the quick, drastic weight loss stories of low-carb dieters. However, there is also prolonged (i.e. more than the first few weeks) weight loss. This prolonged weight loss in low-carb/high-protein diets is also due to ketosis-induced appetite suppression.

Ketosis is a metabolic process that, in simplest terms, is the break-down of fat as fuel. Now, doesn't that sound great? By increasing protein and reducing carbohydrate intake we can make our body break down fat as fuel. Finally, a way to make our body use up those love handles, spare tires and thunder thighs as fuel. This is great in theory; however, excessive or prolonged ketosis in the body has negative results — such as elevated levels of nonessential fats in the blood stream, dehydration, kidney stones, and osteoporosis.

In the end, how exactly low-carbohydrate diets cause weight loss is uncertain. It is likely that it involves everything we've noted:

water loss, ketosis and caloric restriction. Water loss can cause quick changes in weight, however it is a misleading way to lose weight as it can result in quick weight gain after the diet ceases. Ketosis comes with consequences that may not be worth it. In fact, the Mayo Clinic Women's HealthSource noted in its 2003 October issue that fast weight loss doesn't make the low-carb diet safe.[17] The potential health effects of ketosis (e.g. dehydration, kidney stones, osteoporosis and fatty blood) are extensive and concerning. The third possible cause, caloric restriction, is one we have known about for a long time and is well-known as being effective for weight loss.

In addition, longer diet duration may also be a reason for the success of this diet. This is likely due to the satiety from the higher fat in low-carb diets which seems to keep dieters on this diet longer than other types of diets. These conclusions are supported by current research. A review, by Stanford researchers, on the efficacy and safety of low-carbohydrate diets concluded that people who go on low-carbohydrate diets typically lose weight. However, restricted caloric intake and longer diet duration are the biggest reason why.[18]

Therefore, if the weight loss associated with low-carb diets is possibly a combination of these three causes, some safe and others not, the question remains: Is the weight loss from low-carb diets safe?

As 70 million Americans were at one point limiting their carbohydrate intake without formally dieting,[19] discovering the safety of low-carb diets is very important to our health. Let's investigate the current scientific understanding of this area to date.

Researchers at Stanford collected literature on low-carb diets published between 1966 and 2003. They reviewed 107 diet studies, which involved 3,268 people from around the world. The studies were small and heterogeneous, and varied greatly on carbohydrate and caloric intake, diet duration and participant characteristics. However, all of the studies involved people less than 53 years of age, and no study lasted longer than 90 days. In other words, the researchers found that the information available on older adults and on long-term effects is scarce. Therefore, any conclusions we can make here will only pertain to the use of this diet over 3 months and in adults below the age of 53.

The Stanford researchers' meta-analysis (review of all existing studies) concluded that eating 60 grams or less of carbohydrates a day did cause weight loss. In fact, the greatest weight loss occurred in those who had a lot of weight to lose (highest baseline weight) and those with the lowest caloric intake. The weight loss seen in the low-carb diet was associated with caloric intake restriction and longer diet duration, not with reduced carbohydrate intake. In other words, the diets do cause weight loss but it is not due to carbohydrate restriction. The findings suggest that if you want to lose weight, you should eat fewer calories and do so over a long time period.

Perhaps more importantly, the study looked at some safety measurements of the diet. The researchers found no significant adverse effects on cholesterol, glucose, insulin and blood-pressure levels among participants on the diets. But, as one of the researchers, Bravata, stressed in a press interview, the adverse effects may not have shown up within the short period of the studies.[20] Also, it is very important to realize that losing weight typically leads to an improvement in the levels of these blood health markers, so this could have had an impact on the numbers.

b) Low-Carb versus Low-Fat for Weight Loss

Low fat diets have been around for decades and claimed by many to be the best diet for weight loss. However, for over 20 years, there have been some scientific studies that have showed low-carbohydrate diets produce at least as much weight loss, if not more, than conventional energy-restricted, low fat diets.

More recently, there have been a small number of studies looking at low-carbohydrate diets that may enlighten us as to whether a low-carbohydrate or a low-fat diet is best for weight loss.

1) A randomized control trial, involving 63 obese men and women, had one group use the Atkins New Diet Revolution book diet (e.g. low-carbohydrate/high fat/high-protein) and the other group use an energy restrictioned low fat (25% of energy) diet. After 6 months on the diets the low-carbohydrate/high-fat/high-protein diet (i.e. Atkins diet) resulted in greater weight loss than the conventional low energy/low fat diet. However, after on year the low-carb diet did not result in significantly more weight loss than the low fat diet.[21]

2) A study randomly assigned 53 obese females to one of two diets for 6 months. Diet one had no caloric restrictions but, very low in carbohydrates, which is similar to the low-carb diet we've been discussing. Diet two was energy-restricted and low in fat, which is similar to the traditional low fat diet. After 6 months the low-carbohydrate group had lost more weight.[22]

These two studies state that low-carbohydrate diets are more effective for short-term weight loss. However, they also point out that in the long-run the traditional low-fat diet is just as effective. Therefore, since good dietary practices should be practiced permanently it would appear that a low-fat diet is better as it appears to have better long-term benefits.

These two studies state that low carb diets are more effective for short-term weight loss. However, they also point out that in the long-run the traditional low-fat diet is just as effective for weight-loss.

c) Low-Carb for Low Weight?

What a great question! Do low-carb diets cause you to have a lower weight? Let's have science answer this question. A meta-analysis (i.e. a critical review of all the scientific literature on the topic) on low-carbohydrate diets concluded that there is insufficient evidence to make recommendations for, or against, the use of low-carbohydrate diets. They continued to state that "among the published studies, participant weight loss while using low-carbohydrate diets was principally associated with decreased caloric intake and increased diet duration but not with reduced carbohydrate content."[23]

Perhaps the confusion behind the effectiveness of low carbohydrate diets to cause weight loss is due to the lack of definition of a carbohydrate. Not all carbohydrates are created equal. There are both simple and complex carbohydrates - each of which has a very different effect on the body.

As discussed in more detail later in this book, the consumption of high glycemic foods, also known as simple or bad carbohydrates, promotes the storage of excess energy as fat and promotes frequent eating. Thus simple carbohydrates may be associated, in part, with obesity.

However, complex carbohydrates may have a very different effect. In fact, research supports the use of complex carbohydrates for weight loss. Complex carbohydrate consumption actually boosts metabolism. It is well known that foods rich in complex carbohydrates stimulate the thyroid gland resulting in more efficient calorie burning. In other words, if you eat complex carbs, you have more efficient calorie burning or weight loss. For example, in 2003, a study presented at the *Experimental Biology* meeting in California revealed that oatmeal, a commonly consumed carbohydrate, can play a role in preventing childhood obesity.[24] Therefore, evidence suggests that it is quite possible that it is not "carbohydrates" that are making us fat. But a diet high in complex carbohydrates is a recipe for weight loss.

So, does a low-carbohydrate diet cause weight loss? Scientifically it appears that this cannot be conclusively confirmed. However, it does appear that a diet low in simple carbohydrates would promote a healthier weight.

Let's take a look at the other possibility. Do anti-carb or extremely low–carb diets cause weight gain? According to one researcher: "Although many environmental factors promote a positive energy balance, it is clear that the consumption of a low-carbohydrate, high-fat diet increases the likelihood of weight gain. Data on sucrose intake, in relation to metabolism and weight gain, do not associate high consumption of sucrose with the prevalence of obesity. The evidence supports the current dietary guidelines for reducing fat intake. However, the effect of a carbohydrate's source, class and form (solid or liquid) on body weight control requires further consideration"[25] Therefore, we know that carbohydrate consumption is not directly linked with obesity. And, that science does suggest that it is possible that low-carbohydrate, high-fat diets increase the likelihood of weight gain.

All in all, it appears that according to North Americans, the stories in low-carbohydrate diet books, the thousands of copies sold, and the success of low-carbohydrate food products, citizens think low-carb diets are effective. According to science we know that simple carbohydrates are likely promoters of weight gain, but complex carbohydrates are likely promoters of a more balanced, healthy weight. Therefore, science says that the good, complex carbohydrates seem to be the scientific weight loss winner. As for the scientists…well, the scientists do not all agree.

d) The Truth about Weight Loss and Dieting

Based on our current scientific knowledge there is only one certain thing about weight loss and dieting. After all the science is reviewed, there is only one known way to safely and effectively lose weight. The only healthy and sustainable way to lose weight is a caloric deficit of 500kcal/day. To explain, one pound of fat is 3,500 calories. To loose one pound a week (e.g. seven days), the amount noted historically to be safe and sustainable, there needs to be a 500 calorie deficit per day.

Why are low calorie diets so effective at weight loss? Low calorie diets, such as the conventional Japanese diet have been shown to be useful in weight reduction. Low calorie foods are conventionally high in fibre thereby the mastication (e.g. chewing) required increases and, there is enhancement of satiation. In other words you tend to be more satisfied when you have to chew your food more.

Good, or complex carbohydrates have a lower energy density (i.e. are low in calories) and have a greater satiety capacity. Therefore, if lower calorie consumption is the only healthy and sustainable way to lose weight, than a diet that promotes the intake of complex carbohydrate foods is likely a diet that causes humans to limit consumption of calories. In other words, a diet high in good carbs may be one that causes weight loss.[26]

Perhaps more importantly, a healthy weight is part of a healthy lifestyle that includes exercise, and good mental health. Yes, your mental health can affect your weight. Here's an interesting piece of physiology - when under stress, the body reacts by storing fat. Stress can cause the body to release a hormone, cortisol. Cortisol stimulates the appetite and the body to store fat for a future emergency. Perhaps stress is the reason we are an overweight society, as our lifestyles are very stressful. In fact, it has been estimated that about 1/3 of visits to primary care physicians are for stress related problems.[27] Therefore, reducing stress is a good part of a good weight loss program. Great ways to reduce stress include exercising, yoga, meditation and taking the time to breathe deeply each hour.

e) The Goods on Low-Carb Diets

The scientific debate about the effectiveness and benefits of low-carbohydrate diets is far from over. As research notes, there are some serious flaws and some promising theories with low-carbohydrate diets. Some researchers adamantly support these diets. For example, Volek and Westman made it clear in their comment in the November 2002 issue of the *Cleveland Clinical Journal of Medicine* that very low-carbohydrate diets merit further investigation and that criticisms of such diets appear to lack evidence.[28]

On the other hand, some researchers support the use of good carbohydrates and the elimination of the bad carbohydrates. DS Ludwig, in a 2003 edition of *Lipids,* notes that the rates of overweight and obese people has risen in developed countries since the 1960s despite public health efforts to encourage reduced fat intake and increased physical activity. Therefore, Ludwig argues for the utility of low glycemic index diets (i.e. diets that are high in good, complex carbohydrates and low in bad, simple carbohydrates) in the prevention and treatment of obesity and related complications.[29]

Therefore, it appears that the debate on low-carbohydrate diets may be far from over. We can generally conclude that a diet low in bad or simple carbohydrates is a good idea as it appears to be supported by scientists, science and stories by the North American public. As for the marketed low-carbohydrate/high-fat diets, it appears that, to date, we can't conclude how successful they will be at causing weight loss.

In our quest to find a healthy diet in the wake of the low-carb craze it is important to look deeper in the high-protein/ low-carbohydrate diet. Firstly, let's investigate the history of low-carb, the facts on fats, proteins and carbohydrates. Then, let's determine what a good diet is through an investigation of respected diets of our time. Come on, let our quest begin.

Chapter 2:
Foundation of the
High-Protein / Low-Carb Diet

To be able to discuss and uncover the truth about carbohydrates, protein, fat in our quest to find a good diet, we need to fully understand the high-protein/low-carbohydrate diet.

a) History of the Low-Carb Diet

Earlier I suggested that the low-carbohydrate diet started in 1972 with Dr. Atkins' book, *The New Diet Revolution*. However some suggest that the notion of a low-carbohydrate diet started almost a century earlier. In 1864, William Banting published his own personal experience with a low-carbohydrate diet in *Letter on Corpulence*. Banting, an overweight undertaker, thought he was losing his hearing. When he visited his doctor, Dr. Harvey, he was instructed to ban sugar, starch, beer and potatoes from his diet as his obesity was pressing on his inner ear, affecting his hearing. After losing 100 pounds on this low-carbohydrate diet, Banting published his experiences in his letter. Little did he know that he would be the first guinea pig of the low-carb experience nor that his little experimental diet would become a dietary phenomenon a little more than a century later. With this letter he started the debate of whether it is what you eat or how much you eat that matters. This is a debate that still rages.

The question of the quantity of food consumed was soon questioned again. In the late 1800s Wilbur Atwater, a chemist, created the measurement of a calorie. This was calculated by burning food in a calorimeter (i.e. a small oven) and measuring the amount of heat it produced. Since the human body works like an oven burning food for energy, the measurement of a calorie became a useful way to measure the amount of energy we eat. Other scientists later calculated the amount of heat created in the human body during various activities and, were able to estimate how many calories are used. Now there was an equation to calculate the total energy put into the body and the total energy used. This is known as the energy balance theory. The concept was that if you or eat more calories than you burn, you will gain weight. The vice versa will cause weight loss. So began the argument that weight is determined by how much we eat.

However, not everyone believes that all calories are created equally. As Banting noted in his letter, what he ate might have made more of a difference on his fat cells than how much he ate. Banting believed that eating carbohydrates encouraged his fat cells to grow. Low-carb theorists believe that the kind of calorie consumed determines your hormonal response to the food, and therefore, the way you respond to certain foods. This theory fuels the argument that not all calories are created equally, arguing that carbohydrates may be worse than other forms of food in causing fat accumulation. This theory led to many intriguing questions about varying diets around the world and their effects on health and weight.

Populations around the world are known for varying diets. For example, take a stroll down the restaurant section of a large town near you. There are Italian, Chinese, Greek, Asian and North American type restaurants. Now many of us may just think that the difference is in the seasonings. However, a closer look identifies that there are differences in the types of meat, amount of pastas and breads and types of vegetables in the typical cuisine of these restaurants. The diet of these populations varies in the amount of protein and carbohydrates that they eat. However, there is more science to noting variances in population diets than a stroll down the street.

In 1926, an explorer named Stefansson did a number of exhibitions in the Arctic where he consumed the high meat and fat diet of the Inuits. Stefansson noted that the Inuits were in great health despite the proposed theory that a high fat diet could cause hardenings of the arteries and kidney problems. His intrigue of this controversial observation was shared by a number of physicians who put him through a number of examinations. The results were published in the *Journal of the American Medical Association.*[30]

They stated that an all meat and protein diet, as eaten by the Inuits, appears to have no harmful health effects. However, this data should not be taken as proof that a North American diet high in meat will have no harmful effects. The type of meat and fat consumed by the Inuits is very different than that of the typical North American. Inuits eat a lot of fish, which is lower in saturated fats and high in polyunsaturated fats, also known as omega-3 fatty acids. North Americans tend to eat a lot of beef and other red meats which are high in saturated fat and cholesterol. Not all fats are created equal. And, as such the question of what we eat versus how much we eat grew more intriguing.

Stefansson questioned the high fat diet of the Inuit yet it was not until the 1950s that scientists confirmed that a high fat diet is bad for the heart. Ancel Keys was a scientist who researched the relationship between heart disease and diet. Keys and his colleagues from seven countries posed the hypothesis that differences in the frequency of heart attacks and strokes between different populations would somehow be related to the physical characteristics and lifestyles of these people. They hypothesized that differences in the composition of the diet, particularly fats, would play a key role.

So, the scientists set out to test their hypothesis. The *Keys' Seven Countries Study*,[31] started with surveys completed by populations of men, ages 40-59, in eighteen areas of seven countries, for 12 years (1958 to 1970). The Keys' Seven Countries Study was state of the art for its time. It was a comparison study of populations, across a wide range of diet, risk and disease experience and, was the first to explore associations among diet, risk and disease in contrasting populations. Such studies are highly respected as good indicators of population trends despite some faults in its research methods.

This extensive study concluded that cholesterol is a cause of heart disease and that saturated fat can cause cholesterol levels to rise.[32] These results caused a large change in societal perception of fat and, were the beginning of our fat phobia that swept the continent in the 1970s and 1980s. People began to fear fat.

The fat phobia of the eighties was fueled by a growing body of scientific studies indicating that a diet high in fat was associated with an increased risk of disease. It was even backed by a bureaucratic division in the United States, called the National Cholesterol Education Program. As the public tried to eliminate fat from their diets by cutting out items such as dairy and meat, they avoided most sources of protein. To appease their fat and protein deficient diets North Americans filled up on carbohydrates. The tables turned and North American's started to consume up to 50% of their diet as carbohydrates. The term low-fat became the hottest marketing term of the nation. Low-fat foods were the hit of the time. This fat phobic wave in dietary change over-shadowed the launch of the low-carbohydrate theory of the now best known low-carbohydrate theorist, Dr. Atkins.

In 1972, the creator of the most successful commercial low-carb diet, Dr. Atkins, released *The New Diet Revolution.* Despite its supporting science and exciting twist to conventional thinking, its launch was overshadowed by the fat phobia of the times. The momentum of the fat phobia created by the media was far too great for the unique diet perspective of the low-carb theorist. Dr. Atkins' philosophy of dieting never really caught on. Why has it caught on now? Well, by the late 1990s, the public realized that low fat diets were not working. As a society, we are getting fatter. In fact, the percentage of Americans who are overweight has increased 10% in the last decade. Not to mention the epidemic of diabetes we are facing which some suggest may be due to our love for carbohydrates and our inability to keep our weight in check. As the public has become frustrated with low fat diets, the desire for a new diet trend grew and now we see the emergence of the new wave of dieting – 'the low-carb lifestyle'.

Today, no matter where you look there are low-carb advertisements, articles and products. In fact, even some non-food products are advertising they are carb-free, as the concept of no-carbs has caught everyone's attention. Just the other day the billboard off the freeway showed the most recent motorcycle and its noted selling features included its sleek design, great motor power and that is was carb-free. The craze has grabbed hold of the nation. The nation is divided by those who are for the diet, and those who oppose it. Who is right? It is hard to know as the messages are many and confusing. The truth is not easy to see. Perhaps it is not so much of who is right as surveys suggest that almost every North American is at some level becoming conscious of the amount of carbohydrates they consume. And, the more conscious we are of our food, the less we tend to eat. Ultimately, there is a great need to understand carbohydrates, and there is a great need to know the truth about carbohydrates.

b) The Founding Theories of the High-Protein/Low-Carb Diet

To understand the low-carb phenomenon we need to start with the original low-carb diet. Let's investigate the founding theories of the high-protein/low-carbohydrate diet as described in Dr. Robert Atkins', *Atkins for Life*.[33] This high protein /low-carbohydrate dietary theory is founded on a well balanced diet that cuts out white, processed carbohydrates and encourages protein consumption. As most North Americans have a low consumption of protein, encouraging increased protein consumption is not a bad suggestion, particularly when 'high-quality' sources of protein such as nuts, fish and, soy are encouraged as protein sources. However, most typical North American protein sources are laced with saturated fat and cholesterol. Just think about our typical fast-and-easy meals: hamburgers, sausages and hotdogs. Consumption of these types of protein leads to a diet that is high in bad fat which is not part of a healthy, balanced diet. Despite confusion from current media messaging, the wraps and salads that are high in bacon, cheese and beef are also sources of bad fat. The consumption of high fat sources of protein is limited in the Atkin's dietary theory.

The high-protein/low–carbohydrate diet as described in *Atkins for Life*, goes beyond the request to increase protein consumption and, advises a restriction in carbohydrate consumption. The suggestion to cut out white, processed carbohydrates is good nutritional advice. We are a society that loves white bread, candy and white pasta. These white carbohydrate foods have evolved into a major part of our daily diets over the past two decades. As we have attempted to cut sources of fat from our diet we've filled the fat gap with carbohydrates. Over consumption of white/processed carbohydrates can result in limited consumption of more valuable foods such as fruits and vegetables and good quality protein. Over consumption of white/processed carbohydrates may also cause weight gain. Also, scientists have found links between eating a lot of carbohydrates and poor health conditions such as reduced immune function,[34,35] type II diabetes,[36] and epileptic seizures in children.[37] Therefore, it appears that suggesting a limitation on white/processed carbohydrates is good nutritional advice.

As we have altered our diets over the last decade we've allowed ourselves to greatly rely on carbohydrates, most of them are highly processed as we demand on-the-go, convenient foods. Simply think about the increase in sales of potato chips, crackers, microwave dinners and grain-based snack bars. Therefore, the suggestion in the diet theory, by Dr. Atkins, to reduce carbohydrate consumption is a good idea.

However, it's important to note that not all carbohydrates are equal. In scientific studies, weight gain was inversely associated with the intake of high-fiber, whole-grain foods but positively related to the intake of refined-grain foods.[38] This suggests that not all carbohydrates are created equal, and that they may play a role in obesity. Followers of this original low-carb diet, as described by Dr. Atkins, tend to miss these important facts: 1) Not all carbohydrates are created equal; 2) Carbohydrates may play a role in weight loss.

The founding theories of the original low-carb diet are to reduce consumption of carbohydrates and increase consumption of protein while restricting large consumption of fatty foods. As with all things, this is easier said than done. Therefore, a diet timeline was also created to help dieters learn this new way of eating. Nothing can happen over night. We cannot expect ourselves to make sustainable changes to our diets quickly. All habits take time to change. Particularly our dietary habits as they are reflective of our parents' diets, behaviors and societal influences. Food choices are an entrenched habit that can be difficult to change.

c) The Original Low-Carb Diet Timeline

Changing your diet cannot happen over night. You need to train yourself to crave different foods, buy different items at the grocery store and consume a different diet. In *Atkins for Life,* it is suggested that one starts the diet with a two week 'Induction' phase. In this phase you are requested to seek out high quality protein sources and to limit your Net Carbs (i.e. the carbohydrates that are not fibre or sugar alcohols) to 20 grams a day. Why do they eliminate the fibre and sugar alcohol from the counting system? Well, as we noted earlier, not all carbs are created equally. Fibre is generally undigested in the body. Hence, the advertisements from high fibre cereals that fibre is like the plumber of your intestines – it pushes through everything, cleaning your 'pipes' out. The reason the Atkin's diet chooses to subtract sugar alcohols is because they contain about half of the calories as their carbohydrate counterparts. Also, they are converted to glucose more slowly, thereby requiring little or no insulin to be metabolized and don't cause sudden increases in blood sugar. In other words, sugar alcohols cause less of a reaction in your body and are lower in calories than sugar, therefore sugar alcohols are not calculated the same as other carbohydrates in the Net Carb calculation.

It is important to realize that Net Carbs are not the actual number of carbohydrates as they appear on the nutritional panel of food products. Only Atkins' products indicate the Net Carbs on their packaging. Therefore, it is important to understand that in the 'Induction' phase when you are only to eat 20 grams of carbohydrates that it is Net Carbs that they are talking about. Therefore, if you are attempting to determine the Net Carbs of a traditional food product from the nutritional panel you need to start with the total carbohydrates and subtract the fibre. This can be a little helpful in estimating the Net Carbs. But, remember that this number is still inflated as you have yet to subtract the sugar alcohol, which unfortunately we can't determine without a chemistry set in the store aisles. A list of sugar alcohols are noted in Table 1. And, since we all do not tend to carry chemistry sets in our purses and backpacks, a list of common food sources of sugar alcohols is available in Table 2.

All in all, one most important point to realize is that the recommended Net Carbs in the Induction phase, or first phase of the Atkin's diet, is far less carbohydrates than one typically eats in a classic North American diet. Why does the Atkin's diet require such a drastic reduction in carbohydrates? One suggested reason for this harsh carbohydrate restriction is that it challenges you to identify all the sources of carbohydrates in your diet. Once you identify these sources you remove them and seek out alternatives. This drastic and harsh technique to get one to change their dietary choices is an interesting tool to make people change. However, whether such drastic changes are healthy or helpful in making long term positive changes in dietary choices is not certain. Perhaps the more questionable aspect of the Induction phase approach is that some people stay on this first phase, never moving onto phase two. This is not advised by the original high protein/low-carbohydrate diet theorists as carbohydrates are a vital part of our diets and a lack of carbohydrates has many negative biological effects including increased risk of cardiovascular and renal disease. The dangers of staying on the Induction Phase, a very low-carbohydrate phase, or a diet that is low in carbohydrate consumption will be discussed in more detail in Chapter 4.

The desire of North Americans to stay on the Induction Phase is puzzling. It may be the desire to have quick results. However, it is not healthy as one young women's mother noted to me at a recent seminar on carbohydrates. Her daughter looked grey, lethargic and depressed. Her mother was concerned that it was her insistence to stay on the Induction Phase beyond the recommended two weeks that was causing these effects. As she learned, and as will you, carbohydrates are an important part of a healthy diet. In fact, this phase approach of the Atkin's diet shows us just how important carbohydrates are by quickly reintroducing them in phase 2.

The second phase in *Atkins for Life* is called the Ongoing Weight Loss stage. This stage suggests that high value carbohydrates be added back into the diet while still trying to focus on high quality protein sources. These include whole grain pastas, cereals, breads and most fruits and vegetables. This second phase adds about 5 Net Carbs more each week for a total of 25 Net Carbs.

The interesting point to realize is that the total number of carbohydrates that you are consuming increases as the week's progress. Why? The types of foods added in phase two are high in fibre, and therefore have a low Net Carb count, thereby allowing you to increase your total carbohydrate intake. This is important because carbohydrates are our fuel. Our bodies simply cannot function without carbohydrates. Many who try this diet, in fact, cannot complete the two weeks of the first phase. They find they are like a car without gas. They cannot function properly and they lack energy. This is what the man at the seminar mentioned – feeling lethargic. This is because we need carbohydrates. It's our gas - our fuel. That is why the second phase brings back in these high fibre carbohydrates, or soon to be known as 'good carbs'.

As the diet progresses, more high fibre, high nutritional value carbohydrates are added in with hope that the phases taught us to recognize where carbohydrates are in our diet, and how there are other foods to eat instead. To learn more about carbohydrates and where they are in our diet, see Chapter 3.

There are four phases in total to the *Atkins for Life* diet. For each phase of the Atkins diet there are a hundred stories from people experiencing miraculous weight loss. However, do we really understand what happens to our bodies on a high protein/

low-carbohydrate diet? Or, worse on an anti-carb diet? Do we understand how they work? Do high protein/low-carbohydrate diets cause weight loss? There are so many questions - so many messages from the media and society. What is the truth? We need to understand the types of diets we are using so we can live healthy with less obesity. It is vital for the health of North American's that we uncover the truth about diets, and the truth about carbs.

Table 1: A List of Sugar Alcohols

Xylitol	Isomalt
Maltitol	Lactitol
Sorbitol	Erythritol
Mannitol	Hydrogenated starch hydrolysales

Table 2: Common Foods that can contain Sugar Alcohols

Chewing gum	Soft drinks	Syrups
Cookies	Throat lozenges	Sauces
Hard candy	Toothpaste	Mouthwash

d) Other Low-Carb Diets

Most of our discussion has focused on the most popular of late, low-carbohydrate diet, the Atkins diet. However, there are many other low-carbohydrate diets on the market in the twenty-first century. The next two most popular of these diets, being the Zone diet and, the South Beach Diet. Are these any better than the Atkin's diet? Millions of copies of the South Beach and The Zone diet sell annually. Store aisles are full of products promoted to be part of the low-carb lifestyle. However, one would hope that after all the yo-yo diets we've encountered in North America in the last few decades that we would know that just because something sells, does not mean it works. For example, the multi-million dollar success of the South Beach diet may be associated with the million dollar spend by its publishing company to promote it, opposed to the success of the diet itself. Let's quickly explain the main theory of these two diets and the strength of their science.

The Zone diet is a diet that is supposed to be 40% carbohydrates, 30% protein and 30% fat. It advocates sparing use of starches and grains. The decrease in carbohydrate consumption classifies this diet as low-carb. In an interesting scientific review, Cheuvront highlights some of the main features and faults of the Zone diet. It is thought to promote better insulin to glucagon ratios. A reduction in this ratio is thought to improve eicosanoid metabolism thereby resulting in an improved immune function thereby reducing the risk of chronic disease. To date, there is little scientific support for the connections made between diet, eicosanoid metabolism and disease. Some scientists have even questioned it's efficacy as a diet.[39] The Zone diet offers a slightly different perspective on low-carb dieting; however, its promoted health benefits and ability to cause weight loss are questioned by some scientific studies. This diet is a bit difficult to critique as it has both positives and negatives. Firstly, its 40:30:30 concept appears to encourage a well balanced diet from a variety of food sources. This is a good idea as there are so many different nutri-ents needed by the body for optimal health; it is a good idea to eat a variety of food types to ensure adequate consumption of all needed nutrients. Also, its encouragement to consume more omega-3 fatty acids is a great idea as we know these fats are essential to our health and tend to be lacking from the North American diet.

On the negative side, this diet was created as a heart healthy "drug", according to Sears, not as a lose-weight diet. Therefore, it may not be an effective way for obese North Americans to lose needed weight effectively. Since the Zone diet is fairly close to the Mediterranean diet, one of the healthiest diets of our time, it does not have many aspects to criticize. However, this diet is a bit out of date and it may be worth looking into Sears' more recent work.

The South Beach diet on the other hand, is also a low-carb diet but is more complicated than the Zone diet. In general, the South Beach diet contains a similar 3 part dieting stage as Atkins. It encourages more protein and less carbohydrate consumption. The aspect of the South Beach diet that sets it apart from the others is a few questionable points that raise question to the science and effectiveness of it.

Firstly, the book appears to poorly divide the fats. The South Beach diet appears to highly discourage consumption of any form of saturated fat. Yet, the saturated fat in plant oils is not a great concern, and one saturated fat, stearic acid, found in butter may actually be beneficial. This leads us to the recommendation in South Beach to use margarine, which is full of trans fat, the worst fat of all. Not to mention, the suggestion to eat French fries over a baked potato. Thanks to the section on fat in this manuscript, we all know that margarine is a bad idea, as are fried foods. It appears that the South Beach diet is out of date in its theories on fats.

Secondly, the South Beach diet recommends aspartame as a low calorie sweetener. This is a poor recommendation as some scientific studies have raised concern that aspartame may be a neurotoxin. However, as the use of low calorie sweeteners in a diet may contribute to weight reduction,[40] it is worth noting Stevia. Stevia is a natural herb that tastes sweet; however, contains no carbohydrates or calories because it is not a sugar. It has been used in North America by diabetics for many years as it does not raise their blood glucose levels. Traditionally, it has been used in South America, and is currently used as a food additive in Japan and has been for 3 decades without adverse reactions.

Therefore, it appears that the South Beach diet lacks some recent research and theories. As for the Zone diet, its fundamentals are promising but may not be an effective weight loss diet, as it was not originally designed to be one.

e.) Health Effects of Low-Carb Diets

The health effects of low-carb diets has been debated. Two studies comparing low-carb diets to low-fat diets that were discussed earlier will be used here as they note some intersting health effects.

1) A randomized control trial, involving 63 obese men and women, had one group use the Atkins New Diet Revolution book diet (e.g. low-carbohydrate/high-fat/high-protein) and the other group used an energy restricted low fat (25% of energy) diet. After 6 months on the diets the low-carbohydrate/high-fat/high-protein diet (i.e. Atkins-like diet) resulted in greater weight loss than the conventional low energy/low fat diet. However, after one year, the low-carb diet did not result in significantly more weight loss than the low fat diet. Interestingly, the subjects on the low-carbohydrate diet had greater increases in HDL cholesterol and greater falls in serum triglycerides.[41]

2) A study randomly assigned 53 obese females to one of two diets for 6 months. Diet one had no caloric restictions but, very low in carbohydrates, which is similar to the low-carb diet we've been discussing. Diet two was energy-restricted and low in fat, which is similar to the traditional low-fat diet. After 6 months the low-carbohydrate group had lost more weight. Both groups improved their blood pressure, lipids, fasting glucose and fasting glucose and insulin.[42]

These two studies raise some concerns about the effects of low-carb diets on disease risk factors. Although study one does show a decrease in triglycerides and an increase in HDL, which are thought to be signs of healthy hearts. However, in terms of overall cardiovascular health, ketosis, mobilized fat into the blood stream making it more thick and less fluid, which is not a heart healthy effect. It is important to realize that there are over 200 risk factors for heart disease. Of those, there are many that can be measured from the blood: LDL, HDL, TGs, blood pressure, C-reactive protein, homocysteine, fibrinogen, lipoprotein, and more. Also, we need to remember that the effects of diet take a number of weeks to affect some of these blood levels. Therefore, we are unable to determine if the effect of the low-carb diet on the blood levels of the subjects in these short term studies is a true reflection of the effect of this diet on their cardiovascular health.

As one last point, the diets used in the scientific research studies investigated here are highly controlled and are not necessarily like the low-carb, or anti-carb diets used by North Americans in everyday life. Under the research study conditions, fast food drive-thrus, deep-fried foods, and high bad fat foods are not encouraged or used as freely by the general population. These diets generally are healthier low-carb diets than the American low-carb, high-fat diet. Thus, we cannot reasonably assume that the blood levels noted in the studies above can indicate the cardiovascular safety of the general population's American low-carb diet. Adverse effects of long term increases in protein and saturated fat intake are well known to be of great concern.[43] A diet high in saturated fat is well known to be associated with heart disease. The high blood fat levels caused by ketosis, challenges the safety of the low-carb diet in terms of cardiovascular health. This concern of the effect of low-carbohydrate diets on cardiovascular and on diabetic risk factors has been echoed by the scientific community;[44,45] as the medical associations and physicians have expressed concerns that the low-carb diet is high in fat and may lead to kidney, liver problems and other health risks.

Chapter 3:
Truth about Carbs

About 72% of Canadians say they're aware of the terms "good carbs" and "bad carbs" but only 11% believe they understand the differences.[46] There are over 3/4 of us who do not fully understand what a good carb and a bad carb is. As carbohydrates are a major player in our metabolism it is vital that we figure this out.

Carbohydrates are perhaps, the most important player in our energy system. A diet that lacks carbohydrates is like a car that lacks gas. Carbohydrates are our fuel. Without fuel your car nor your body runs properly.

The United States Food Pyramid and the Canadian Food Guide recommend that about 55% of our dietary energy come from carbohydrates. Currently, in Canada, only 45% of Canadians' dietary energy comes from carbohydrates.[47] Therefore, there is cross-border accord that carbohydrates are an important part of our diets and that we are in fact eating fewer carbohydrates than we are recommended too.

What is a carbohydrate? The simple answer is that a carbohydrate is sugar. Therefore, candy, pop, fruits, vegetables, juices, breads, pastas, rice, grains, nuts, legumes, and dairy all contain carbohydrates.

Carbohydrates come in a variety of forms. To keep it uncomplicated, for the sake of this discussion, there are two types of carbohydrates: complex and simple. They are exactly as they sound. A complex carbohydrate, such as fibre, has many interlocking chains of sugar. Examples of complex carbohydrates include bran, beans, whole wheat bread, and asparagus. A simple carbohydrate, such as white sugar, is only a few sugars linked together. Examples of a simple carbohydrate include candy, pop, berries and white bread. See Table 3.

The metabolism of carbohydrates is both complicated and straightforward. It is complicated as carbohydrates come in a variety of forms (i.e. some simple and some complex) and their metabolism involves a complicated pathway called glycolysis. Carbohydrate metabolism is straightforward as its end results are only carbon dioxide, water and energy.

Table 3: Carbohydrate Types and Examples

Good Carbs	Bad Carbs
Complex	Simple
Starch, glycogen, disaccharides	Monosaccharides
Fibre	Sugar
Whole wheat bread, bran, celery, broccoli, etc.	Candy, white bread, pop, fruit, etc.

a) Digestion of Dietary Carbohydrates

Our diets contain carbohydrates in simple (e.g. white sugar) and complex forms (e.g. fibre). Simple forms of carbohydrates are those that taste sweet, and scientifically are called monosaccharides. Complex forms of carbohydrates include

44

disaccharides, starch (amylose and amylopectin) and glycogen. The most complex carbohydrate, cellulose (fibre), is not digested.

Undigested carbohydrate may be in a separate league. If there are good and bad carbs, then undigested carbohydrates, such as fibre, should be called great carbs. Fibre is a great way to improve the health of your intestines as this undigested material is like a street sweeper – fibre helps keep stuff moving through the intestinal tubes thereby improving the health of your gut.

Carbohydrate digestion is really quite simple. The carbohydrates that start in our mouths have to eventually get into every cell of our body. To do this, the foods we eat have to be digested, or broken down into small pieces so we can absorb them.

The first step in the digestion of carbohydrates is the conversion of complex carbohydrates into smaller, simpler ones. Smaller forms of carbohydrates are easier to absorb, (i.e. transport across the intestinal wall and deliver to the tissues that use them as fuel). The first step begins in the mouth. Let's use an example to explain this process. Imagine eating a piece of bread. This piece of bread is complicated. By looking at it, you can see that there are many vertical and horizontal layers that create bubbles of air in the bread. Let's imagine this piece of bread as a dominos game. Start with a straight line of pieces down the middle of the table and expand from there to make more lines of dominos going both north-south and east-west. This is a two dimensional ideal of what carbohydrates look like. See Figure 1 for a visual.

When you eat bread, you put it in your mouth and chew. As you chew, you find the bread is divided into smaller pieces by the teeth. Saliva contains an enzyme, called amylase, which begins the digestion of carbohydrates. This digestion would be the same as breaking all major intersecting corners in our dominos game. If you were to leave that piece of bread in your mouth long enough it turns into a type of paste. That is the amylase helping breakdown the carbohydrates in the bread. Amylase only works in the mouth and the esophagus. It is virtually inactivated by the strong acid of the stomach.

After you swallow, the bread reaches the stomach. Here the stomach acid works like a cat running over your game of dominos, dividing all of the lines of dominos into small groups of 2 to 4 pieces. In other words, once the food has arrived in the stomach, the acid causes acid hydrolysis causing the bread to break up into smaller pieces.

Then, the bread, which is more like a liquid glue at this point, moves to the small intestine where the main carbohydrate enzyme, alpha-amylase, is found. Alpha-amylase is secreted by the pancreas, an organ of the digestive system. Here, the carbohydrates are converted to the simplest form of carbohydrate, monosaccharides (i.e. one saccharide, or the smallest unit of carbohydrate). This is the equivalent of dividing all of your lines of dominos into individual pieces or pairs of pieces. The enzyme in the small intestine that does this is called saccharidase. Saccharides break monosaccharide chains (e.g. multiple dominos together) into single monosaccharides (e.g. single dominos), including maltases, disaccharidases, sucrase, lactase, and trehalase. The net result is the almost complete conversion of digestible carbohydrate to its constituent monosaccharides, (i.e. the smallest form of carbohydrate, or in our example one domino). Now, the bread is completely broken down into sugar.

The resulting sugar, known scientifically as glucose, is transported across the intestinal wall and to the cells that need to use it as fuel. Inside the cell, a process called glycolysis occurs which allows the cell to convert glucose into energy. (See Figure 2) Under normal conditions the cell has oxygen present (i.e. aerobic conditions) and will oxidize glucose into pyruvate. Next, pyruvate is oxidized in the Citric Acid cycle which creates carbon dioxide and water. The carbon dioxide is sent to the lungs to be breathed out and the water is used in the body. Therefore, the body takes sugar and converts it, fairly efficiently, into a large amount of usable energy, called ATP (adenosine triphosphate). ATP is the energy molecule of the body, like gasoline is to your car. As you probably noticed, there is very little by-product of this reaction. The only things created are energy, water and carbon dioxide. Luckily, the only waste product, carbon dioxide, is very easily removed from your body. This is truly clean burning fuel. If only cars would work as efficiently as our body's do, when converting carbohydrates into energy in the presence of oxygen, we'd have less smog.

Now, when the cell has low levels of oxygen, such as when you are riding a bike for a long period of time, the process of glycolysis does not work as cleanly as noted above. Instead, the body will produce lactate. Since lactate is not easily broken down, the cell can fatigue. This is the reason people talk about lactic acid build up in their muscles during a strenuous workout. However, never fear. The body does eventually break down the lactate; as one may recall, the pain of a hard workout seems to subside eventually.

The most important point to remember about carbohydrate metabolism is that under normal conditions when oxygen is present (i.e. aerobic conditions) the only by-products are water and carbon dioxide. Water is always needed in the body, and carbon dioxide is easily removed by the lungs. Carbohydrates are a clean burning fuel and the most efficient source of energy.

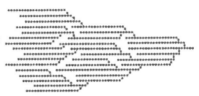

Figure 1: An example of the structure of a carbohydrate.

Figure 2.

Glycolysis – the metabolism of carbohydrates

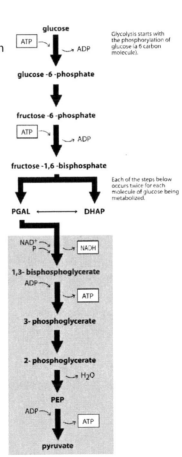

b) Types of Carbohydrates and the Glycemic Index

Not all carbohydrates are created equally. Some carbohydrates are better than others. As we noted earlier, there are both complex carbohydrates and simple carbohydrates. White processed foods are simple carbohydrates. Whole wheat foods are complex carbohydrates. Simple and complex carbohydrates have a different effect on the body.

Recently, there has been hype around the term 'glycemic index'. The glycemic index is a way of measuring the change in blood sugar (i.e. plasma glucose) concentration after a meal. Despite the hype, the glycemic index is nothing new. Scientists have used this measurement for years. One thing to realize is that the glycemic index is different for every food. Each type of food has a different amount and type of carbohydrate in it, therefore each is digested by the body into sugar at a different rate. The glycemic index of a food tells us how our body will respond to consuming it. For example, a piece of white bread will be digested quickly and therefore has a high value on the glycemic index. On the other hand, a whole wheat piece of bread will be digested more slowly by the body and therefore has a lower glycemic index. The faster the rate of digestion of a food the higher the value on the glycemic index. There are examples of glycemic indexes in the back of this manuscript.

High-protein/low-carbohydrate diets use the theory that it is beneficial to reduce the use of simple carbohydrates. This theory is based on the glycemic index. Simple carbohydrates, such as white bread, have a high glycemic index because they can be easily broken down. High-protein/low-carbohydrate diets try to reduce the use of foods that have a high glycemic index as they can have negative effects on the overall health of the body.

49

What happens when you eat a high glycemic index food? Let's use Figure 3 to illustrate. When you eat a high glycemic food, it is a food that can quickly be digested into sugar. Therefore, your body absorbs a large amount of sugar into your blood stream in a very short time. Figure 3 illustrates the effects of simple carbohydrates on the level of sugar in the blood stream. You'll notice in Figure 3 that the simple carbohydrates take your body on a roller coaster ride. There is a very quick increase in blood sugar, and shortly after, a very quick drop in blood sugar concentration.

What causes the blood sugar concentration to drop? The body responds to the digestion of carbohydrates and high levels of sugar in the blood stream by releasing insulin. Insulin is a hormone produced by the pancreas that works in the body to encourage cells to use sugar for energy or to store it as fat. In other words, insulin encourages sugar to be removed from the blood. Insulin is released into the blood stream at a proportional or mirroring rate and concentration to the amount of sugar present. Hence, the even rise and fall of the blood sugar line in Figure 3.

Well, if you can remember that high glycemic index foods cause a high peak in blood sugar, then you will easily remember why such foods are best avoided. It's tough on your body when it goes through this roller coaster ride of high glycemic foods. This is why high protein/low-carbohydrate diets are based on eliminating this type of food from our cuisine. Also, notice that the time it takes for the blood sugar concentration to go from the bottom, to the top, and back down is quite short.

When we eat simple carbohydrates (i.e. high glycemic foods) it causes a quick rise in blood sugar, and a rapid production and release of insulin into the blood stream. This process is so effective it causes almost all of the blood sugar to be pulled out of the blood. The result is low blood sugar. A low level of sugar in your blood stimulates you to think you are hungry. Therefore, you want to eat again. Why? The calories that were consumed when you ate the high glycemic food were not left available for use in the blood stream. Since the large, rapid presence of insulin stimulated the cells to absorb the sugar, the cells were left with more sugar than they can use in a short period of time. When there is excess energy, the body puts it into storage (i.e. fat). Therefore, when you eat high glycemic foods you likely stimulate fat production.

The worse part of this process is what happens to you after the sugar is absorbed by the cells of your body. As your blood sugar level drops, hunger is stimulated. You want to eat again. Even though you have just recently eaten (remember the note of how quick the process is) you end up eating more food. Overall, you end up eating more food than you need to meet your energy needs. Therefore, we can see how simple carbohydrates, or high glycemic index foods, can result in over eating and have been suggested to be associated with obesity.

Complex carbohydrates, on the other hand, are another story. Complex carbohydrates have a low glycemic index because they are harder to digest (i.e. breakdown) into sugar. When you eat a low glycemic index food such as whole wheat bread, your blood sugar rises slowly. The body responds to the slow rise in blood sugar by slowly producing and releasing insulin. This causes the sugar in the blood to gradually move into the body's cells. Unlike the scoffing behavior of the body to a high glycemic food, a low glycemic food is more like spoon feeding. The sugar is available in the blood stream in lower concentrations. Therefore, the cells take little amounts, like spoonfuls of sugar at a time, instead of fists full. Since the sugar is slowly broken down by the digestive tract, it means that it slowly absorbs into the blood, and is slowly taken by the body's cells to use as energy. The overall result is that the sugar is available to the cells for a longer duration of time meaning that when you eat a low glycemic food, or complex carbohydrate, your blood sugar level does not drop low enough to stimulate hunger until much later, than if you had eaten a high glycemic food. So, when you eat low glycemic foods or complex carbohydrates you eat less often. As you probably noticed the cells do not store the sugar as fat. Therefore, eating low glycemic foods theoretically means less overeating, reduced obesity, and perhaps even weight loss. This suggests that a diet low in simple carbohydrates, such as the high protein/low carbohydrate diets, has some healthy foundation.

However, to practice this theory of good and bad carbohydrates we need to be able to determine the glycemic index of a food. As the glycemic index of a food is not typically found on food labels, there is a great need to simplify how to determine the glycemic index of a food. There are many different glycemic index charts in existence. There is no universal standard for measuring the glycemic index of a food - one reason why glycemic index is not on food labels. Therefore, when using a glycemic index chart be sure to compare it with a few others as they can vary from chart to chart. Try to use glycemic index chart numbers as a ball-park indicator of that food's effect on your blood sugar (i.e. glucose) concentration. You'll find examples of glycemic index charts at the back of this book.

As a simple rule; foods that have a high glycemic index include those that can be easily and quickly converted to sugar in the body. For example, white bread, refined cereals, potatoes, and sugar candy are all items that have a high glycemic index. You can imagine how they need very little cutting or digestion to be made into their smallest form. Further, many of these taste sweet.

Remember that sugar can also come in liquid form. Did you know that the average person consumes 170 pounds of sugar annually? This seems like a large number until you realize that a single can of cola contains 12 teaspoons of sugar. Be careful to watch what you are putting in your mouth - it may contain a lot of simple sugar and cause your body to ride the rollercoaster of high glycemic foods.

As for low glycemic index foods, these are those foods that are complex, grainy and fibrous. Low glycemic index foods are usually more 'whole' foods as they are more close to their natural forms than the processed, high glycemic foods. Therefore, low glycemic foods include whole grain breads, pastas and cereals, fruit and vegetables, and nuts.

As a general rule for any healthy diet, we should all reach for low glycemic foods for better health. Whole grain foods are generally accepted as being good for health. The mechanism by which fibrous foods prevent disease is not yet known. It may be gastrointestinal effects, antioxidants, protection and/or phytoestrogens. Regardless, fibre is taking a firm place in the ideal healthy diet. The United States Food and Drug Administration have approved the use of a health claim on food containing whole-grains. *"Diets high in plant foods are associated with a lower occurrence of coronary heart disease and cancers of the lung, colon, esophagus and stomach."* Also, whole grain foods are a valuable source of nutrients that are lacking in the North American diet, including dietary fiber, B vitamins, vitamin E, zinc, selenium, magnesium and copper.

Of note, some people need to control their insulin levels and therefore should focus more on vegetables than fruit in their diet. Also, some people are allergic to gluten. These people should try to avoid breads and other wheat products.

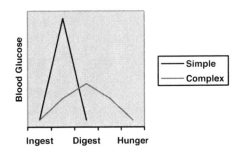

Figure 3: Effects of simple and complex carbohydrates on the level of blood glucose over time.

c) Carbohydrates in Foods

Carbohydrates exist in many forms of foods some of which are better than others. Simple carbohydrates are harder on the body than complex carbohydrates. However, some foods contain both. For example, fruits and vegetables contain both simple and complex carbohydrates. This is obvious as they are sweet tasting (i.e. contain simple carbohydrates) and a known source of dietary fibre (i.e. complex carbohydrates). So, how do you decide if fruits and vegetables are good or bad carbs? One would hope that the answer is obvious. A good carbohydrate is one that has a high nutritional value. A high nutritional value means that a food offers a lot of nutrients that are thought to be helpful to the body. Fruits and vegetables are sources of essential vitamins and minerals and they contain antioxidants and other phytonutrients that are well known health promoters. Therefore, fruits and vegetables contain many helpful and healthy nutrients and therefore are a good carbohydrate and should be part of every healthy diet.

Fruits and vegetables are well known for their ability to reduce the risk of cancer. In *Carcinogenesis*, Thompson et al. 1999 published a study that illustrated the cancer preventing potential of fruits and vegetables[48]. This and many other scientific studies have made convincing arguments that fruits and vegetables do in fact play a role in the prevention of cancer. The argument is so convincing that both Canada and the United States have health claims stating just that. In Canada, "*a diet rich and vegetables and fruit may be associated with a reduced risk of some types of cancer.*" In the United States, "*low fat diets rich in fruits and vegetables may reduce the risk of some types of cancer, a disease associated with many factors.*" These health claims can be found on food products that contain fruits and vegetables in their respective countries.

The secret to vegetables' and fruits' ability to reduce the risk of cancer likely lies in the antioxidants they contain. Antioxidants are like little warriors. They fight the bad compounds in our bodies that cause damage that leads to aging or disease. These bad compounds are called free radicals. Free radicals form naturally in the body and can cause damage to DNA (i.e. the blue prints of our bodies) which can lead to cell death or worse, cell mutation that may lead to cancer. Luckily, antioxidants are great free radical scavengers. And, therefore, fruits and vegetables can save our blue prints from developing errors.

Antioxidants also play a part in the circulatory system. Free radical damage to cells in blood vessels can lead to vessel weakness, or blockage. Such cardiovascular complications can lead to heart attacks and strokes.

Antioxidants are not the only heart friendly fruit and vegetable component. Fibre also plays a role. Fibre can trap cholesterol in the gut in its web-like structure. Fibre can help reduce the amount of cholesterol absorbed from the intestines into the blood stream. Therefore, a diet rich in fibrous fruits and vegetables can be helpful in reducing cholesterol levels. In fact, research has noted many times that diets high in fibre are beneficial for all blood fats.[49] For these and perhaps more reasons, fruits and vegetables are heart healthy foods.

Not that we need another reason to eat fruits and vegetables but, they may also be anti-aging. With age, humans suffer from a degradation of the neuronal system. The neuronal system includes the brain and nerves. As we age, we notice this system can degrade like in age-related dementias, such as Alzheimer's. In 1999, the *Journal of Neuroscience* reported that supplementation with antioxidant rich foods, like fruits and vegetables may reverse the course of neuronal and behavioral aging.[50] Antioxidants found in fruits and vegetables are thought to prevent free radical damage in the brain, thereby preventing damage that occurs naturally with age. Perhaps, the carrot eater truly is the wiser?

All in all, vegetables and fruit contain both good and bad carbs but, because they also contain a power packed punch of antioxidants, they have a very high nutritional value and should be a part of every healthy diet.

Carbohydrates are also in grains and seeds. There is one seed in particular that should be discussed: flax. Have you heard that flax, a source of carbohydrates, can help fight cancer? Flax is a good source of fibre, omega-3 fatty acids, and phytoestrogens. Phytoestrogens are a family of plant compounds (i.e. isoflavones, flavones and lignans). Flaxseed is the richest known source of plant lignans. Accumulating evidence from molecular science, cellular biology, animal studies, and to a limited extent, human clinical trials suggest that phytoestrogens may potentially have health benefits related to heart disease and various cancers.[51,52,53] Researchers have found that flaxseed inhibits human breast cancer growth and metastasis (i.e. the invasive stage of cancer) in mice.[54] Also, flax has been shown to have chemoprotective (i.e. protect healthy cells from negative effects of cancer drugs) effects in animal and cell studies. Some of its effects may be mediated through its influence on hormone production and metabolism.[55] Flax is a natural product with breast cancer prevention potential.

Carbohydrates are in lots of foods. However, we need to identify the total nutritional value of a food before we judge it. Just because it has carbohydrates doesn't mean it is a bad food.

Chapter 4:
Problems with High-Protein/Low-Carb Diets

There is not likely a single person in North America that has not been affected by the extensive media coverage and vast product changes caused by the low-carb phenomenon. Unconciously or concously all of us are now more aware of the carbohydrates we eat.

Research of low-carb dieters has noted an interesting fact – not everyone is doing the same thing. Some low-carb dieters are trying to reduce the amount of white/processed foods they consume. Others are cutting out breads, grains and pastas all together. Another group appears to have cut out carbohydrates entirely from their diets, including fruits and vegetables. This group who is not eating any carbohydrates will be called the 'anti-carb' dieters from here on in.

It is this anti-carb phenomenon that is most concerning. As we have already discovered, the founding theories of the high-protein/low-carb diet is to restrict low value carbohydrates (e.g. white/processed foods), not to cut out fibrous grains, fruits and vegetables. Not all carbohydrates are equal. Carbohydrates are essential to our health – they are our fuel.

Anti-carb dieting results in an increase in the percentage of fat that is consumed because it is hard to fill the hole in the diet where carbohydrates used to be. To fill this carbohydrate hole anit-carb dieters reach for protein. Since one's diet cannot solely be made up of low fat protein sources (nuts, soy, fish) without becoming completely boring, most people start eating other sources of protein such as dairy, beef, chicken and pork which contain higher amounts of fat – and bad fat at that. The anti-carb dieter has missed the facts. They are doing an anti-carb diet that has not been tested for safety or efficacy, and could be danger-ous to their health. Anti-carb dieters do not understand the truth about carbohydrates, protein or fat.

How can the facts of a diet be so misunderstood? To be honest, this is a common occurrence in today's society. The original message of a great concept with tremendous success stories is contorted as it is re-told by various people. For example, scientist or professional tells the story to the reporter. The reporter works on the story and reports it on the news. The person watching the news hears the story and then tells it to their neighbor. The neighbor tells it to the coworker, who tells the story to their sister. The original message, if not super clear and precise, is almost certain to be distorted after so many 're-tellings'. In the instance of the original message of what entails a good diet, it's been distorted into an anti-carb message that has led to an anti-carb trend. The original story from the scientist was a little complicated (i.e. do not eat white and processed carbohydrates and increase good protein sources to lose weight) so, in the re-tellings the story became, don't eat carbs to lose weight.

On the other hand, the anti-carb dieters may be another example of how North American's love to do things to the extreme with the hope that doing more of something will render greater results. In this thinking, cutting out white and processed carbohydrates from your diet is claimed to cause weight loss and, therefore, cutting out all forms of carbohydrates from the diet would be thought to cause faster and greater weight loss. This wishful thinking has not been proven to date, nor is it recommended by nutritionist and medical professionals.

No matter what the reason is for the anti-carb movement in North America, we have created a group of anti-carb dieters. More broadly, our confusion about carbohydrates, protein and fat has created an epidemic of unhealthy eating habits.

In order to better understand carbohydrates, protein and fat, we need to investigate the science behind the high-protein/low-carbohydrate diet. The nutritional science behind high-protein/low-carbohydrate diets is not extensive and at times is controversial. To keep it simple, we'll focus on the three main nutritional concerns surrounding the low-carb diet: high protein consumption, high consumption of bad fat, and the lack of good carbohydrates and essential vitamins and minerals.

a) The Problem with Protein

The arguments surrounding protein and our diets are far reaching. What amount of protein is supposed to be in our diet is a much debated topic. Some scientists and theorists will argue that we were not meant to be meat eaters. That we started on this planet as plant eating animals. These theorists believe that a diet void of meat is best. They agree with the Vegan philosophy of no meat nor animal derived products. Other scientists argue that protein is needed therefore eating meat is an effective way to attain protein. Then again, there are those who think that we

61

were meant to be meat-eaters. They believe that we are carnivores, hunters. Regardless of whether or not we are supposed to eat meat, there is no argument that protein, regardless of source (e.g. meat or plant) is an important part of our diets. Protein is essential in our diets as protein is the major component of our muscles which are vital to our existence. Despite protein's importance in our diets there may be a point where we've had too much protein – a point where protein can have negative consequences.

Perhaps we should start by referring back to the original name of the low-carb diet; the high-protein/low-carbohydrate diet. The term high-protein is perhaps the most confusing aspect to this diet. To a person who eats a lot of meat, a high-protein diet would mean a diet almost completely protein based. For example, dinner would be a 10oz steak and a side of baked beans. However, we are not all the same. To explain, a vegan would see a high-protein diet as being one that quantitatively contain less protein than a meat eater. For example, a high protein dinner to a vegan would be a tofu stir-fry with nuts and beans. If you quantitatively compare the amount of protein in the steak and beans to the tofu stirfry they vary in protein. So, what is high-protein?

In relation to the typical North American diet, does high-protein mean excessive protein, moderate protein or low protein? As the typical North American diet is low in protein (about 20%) we'll assume that to us, the high-protein/low-carbohydrate diet means moderate-protein consumption. In other words, we should increase our protein consumption from 20% to 30% or a bit more. It does not mean to consume 40+% of our diets as protein. However, this is exactly what the anti-carb dieters are doing. The anti-carb dieters are excessively increasing their dietary protein to make up for the lost calories from the removal of carbohydrates from their diet. This excessive increase in protein consumption means that they are really eating a high-protein diet. A high-protein diet has biological consequences.

Now that we understand generally what high-protein means, let's take the time to determine what exact amount would be considered as high-protein, and low-protein consumption? This will help us better understand the studies done on high-protein diets.

Firstly, the typical American diets contain 88-92g (men) and 63-66g (women) protein. A high-protein diet has been noted as consuming about 2g of protein per kilogram of body weight. This means about 160g of protein for an average male (80kg) and 120g of protein for an average female (60kg). Studies using low protein diets have noted 0.8g/kg of protein per day.[56] That would mean that a low protein diet is about 64g/day for an average male (80 kg), and about 48g/day for an average female (60 kg). Therefore, based on scientific studies a high protein diet is 160g for men and 120g for women, and low protein diet is 64g for men and 48g for women.

Too much protein, such as that found in some high-protein diets, particularly the anti-carb diet, can have negative biological effects on the body that can compromise organ function and cause disease. According to George Blackburn, director of the Centre for the Study of Nutrition and Medicine at Boston's Beth Israel Deaconess Medical Center, high protein diets also have annoying side effects including bad breath, constipation, fatigue, nausea, dizziness, irritability, and light-headedness. Protein metabolism and its effects on the body are an important aspect for us to discuss in our quest to understand the truth about carbs.

i) Protein Metabolism

To understand the effects of dietary protein on our bodies we need to be aware of protein metabolism. Firstly, let's investigate protein metabolism. Protein is a complex chain of building blocks. To simplify this investigation, imagine a number of interlocking paper circles, similar to the paper chains that children make as Christmas tree decorations. Each circle represents an amino acid. An amino acid is the smallest unit of protein. They are the building blocks by which proteins are made. The circles of the paper chain, or amino acids, are joined together to form a chain, similarly how amino acids bind together to form a protein. Proteins are not necessarily straight lines like our paper chain. Proteins are more like globs of amino acids, with branching chains and many bonds in three dimensions. So, imagine the paper chain as a heap on the floor. There, now we have an idea of what a protein looks like.

In the body, protein has to be cut by enzymes (i.e. scissors) in order for the building blocks (e.g. amino acids) to be free for use to use to create the proteins we need. To better explain, when protein is consumed our teeth work to break it down into smaller pieces before we swallow. This would be like stepping on our heap of paper chain and breaking it into four or five smaller heaps. Once protein passes through the stomach, it reaches the upper intestine where organs, such as the pancreas, secrete enzymes into the gut to help protein digestion. There are many enzymes involved in protein digestion. Eventually, the enzymes break the protein down into its individual amino acids which can than be absorbed by the body. If these enzymes were to work on our paper chain, they would be like a pair of scissors cutting each chain so that we are left with only unconnected paper circles. The actual process of protein metabolism is not as simple as this Christmas craft. However, it helps us understand what a protein might look like.

Protein metabolism is more complicated than this childhood example. There are by-products and environmental changes involved as well. Protein breakdown, or digestion, creates by-products. One such by-product is called uric acid. High protein diets can result in an increased production of uric acid in the body. Uric acid can cause the formation of small crystals in the joints, usually in the large toe. These crystals cause damage and inflammation known as gout.[57] Gout can be a debilitating condition that causes swelling and pain in the joints.

These by-products of protein metabolism have to be altered and cleared from the body in order to prevent damage that can cause disease such as gout. The liver and kidney are the organs in our bodies that tidy and clean. Extra protein in the diet means that the liver and kidneys have to work very hard. This may speed the progression of disease of these organs, including diabetic renal disease.[58] We also have a national problem of dehydration which challenges the kidneys. North Americans also tend to abuse their liver through over consumption of fatty foods and alcohol. After the fatty food, alcohol and dehydration, the added burden of protein byproducts may be too much for the kidney, a vital organ, to sustain.

Protein metabolism also involves the body's pH, or acid/base balance. Low pH is acidic. High pH is basic. Eating protein causes the body's blood to become acidic. However, the body does not like change. The body always tries to stay the same, a process known as homeostasis. So, when protein is consumed and the

65

blood becomes acidic, the body responds by attempting to counterbalance this acidity. It does this by adding something that is of basic pH to the blood. Calcium is basic, and available to balance the acidic blood. The calcium used in this process comes from, or is pulled from, the muscles and bones.[59] As calcium is a precious mineral in our body, needed for every muscle contraction, teeth strength and bone rigidity this is not an ideal way to use it. The result of pulling calcium from the muscles and bones to counterbalance the acidity of protein consumption can lead to an increased risk of osteoporosis. We'll discuss this more in the next section.

Of note, fruits and vegetables can also cause the blood to be basic. Therefore, consuming fruits and vegetables, when protein is eaten, decreases the need for calcium to be pulled from the bones. Therefore, consuming fruits and vegetables when protein is consumed may reduce the risk of osteoporosis. Perhaps the old fashioned advice of a well balanced diet does have its merits since it appears from this that a diet that has fruits, vegetables and protein is a healthy idea for your bones and muscles.

In general, a diet high in protein can be challenging to the body. Since protein is not a clean burning energy source, its by-products can cause damage such as gout, liver and kidney disease and perhaps even osteoporosis.[60]

ii) Protein and Bones

Have you ever really thought about your bones? Or, what you would be without them? Humans would be heaps of water and cells if it weren't for our bones. We'd be like the big green blob in the Ghost Buster's movie. Our bones are important to us and therefore it is important to understand what may happen to our bones when we eat high amounts of protein.

The effect of high-protein/low-carb diets on bone health is currently a greatly debated topic in the scientific community. Recently, a study reported that high protein diets may boost bone health. Yet, historically, science has suggested that high protein diets are not good for bone health. As mentioned earlier, the amount of protein consumed and the body's calcium levels are related. We noted that eating protein causes the blood to become acidic causing calcium, an alkaline source, to move from the bones to the blood. Therefore, eating protein pulls calcium from the bones. Thus, to date nutritionists and scientists warn of the harm of using a high-protein diet which historically science suggests may promote osteoporosis. Let's take a look at the science to see if we can make a conclusion of our own as to the affect of high-protein/low-carbohydrate diets on bone health.

Historically, science does support the theory that protein consumption is bad for the bones. Scientists have suggested that diets low in protein is good for longevity.[61] These two points suggest that low protein diets are good for your health. Also, another review of the scientific research noted that high protein consumption causes an increase in calcium loss through the urine.[62] This is a bad sign, as calcium loss from the urine suggests a negative flush of calcium from the body. Therefore, it would appear that a diet high in protein forces the body to pull calcium from the muscles and the bones in order to balance the acidity of the blood. With the ever growing number of North Americans developing osteoporosis, this calcium loss from protein consumption is of great concern.

On the other hand, some more recent research is suggesting that the opposite might be true. Perhaps protein consumption does not negatively affect the bones. The *Journal of Clinical Endocrinology and Metabolism*[63] published a study that described how high protein diets may in fact boost bone health by reducing bone re-absorption. This small study of 32 men and women, over the age of 50, randomized the subjects into a high or low protein diet for nine weeks. This short term study also included the recommended 800 milligrams of calcium in the diet. The researchers tested urinary calcium excretion (e.g. a common marker used to determine calcium/bone metabolism) in the two groups. They found no significant difference. In fact, those who increased their dietary protein by an average of 58 grams a day had an increase in bone growth factor and lower levels of markers for bone re-absorption, suggesting that eating lots of protein has a bone healthy effect. In addition, a scientific review of high protein diets reported that high protein diets may not be bad for the bones.[64]

Therefore, it appears that what we have seen is that some say a low protein diet is best for the bones, while others seems to suggest that a high protein diet has bone healthy effects. Thus, the question is, what amount of protein do you have to consume to be bone healthy? Let's look at two studies that noted their dosages for a high and low protein diet. According to the study noted earlier from the Journal of Clinical Endocrinology and Metabolism, consuming a relatively high amount of protein is about 138 g/day for males, and 124 g/day for females (e.g. eating five cans of tuna a day). A low protein diet is 56 g/kg for an average* male and 42 grams per kilogram for an average female (e.g. about a can and a half of tuna a day) according to some studies. This low protein diet was shown to be unhealthy for bones (i.e. lower calcium absorption from the gut and lower bone density).[65] Therefore, it would appear that a diet that had more than 56 g/kg for males and 42 g/kg for females is a good idea. As for an upper limit, it is debatable to what is too much. The high protein diet study above notes a dietary protein intake of double that of the lower protein diet. Likely one should not consume more protein than that. According to North American food guidelines a diet should consist of about one third of its energy from protein.

Why is there such confusion over the effect of protein on the body? As we already know, eating protein causes the body to remove calcium from the bones to reduce the resulting acidic change to the blood. However, protein also affects calcium absorption in the gut (i.e. calcium going into the body). Therefore, protein seems to affect calcium going into the body and calcium coming out. This may explain why scientists have found an increased number of bone turnover markers in the urine of high protein dieters[66] but no net negative loss in bone mass. Perhaps this is the reason there is such confusion. All in all, it appears that the good-old role of thumb that everything in moderation is appropriate for protein consumption when considering bone health.

Another issue that should be noted is that when on a high-protein/low carbohydrate diet, the aim is to lose weight. Weight loss is a factor that one must consider when discussing bone health. Weight loss, as sought out in low-carb diets, is associated with increased bone turnover.[67] It is possible that the induced weight loss in a high-protein/low-carbohydrate diet may itself cause negative effects on bone health.

As you can see, the debate as to whether high, moderate or low protein is best for bone health may be never ending. Which is it, then? High protein or low protein diets for good bones? And, what is the ideal amount of protein for bones? Scientists and nutritionists suggest that a moderate intake of protein is the best choice as it will be beneficial for calcium absorption but will not cause excessive calcium loss from the bones.

Luckily, there is one fact about protein consumption and bone health that we can say with complete confidence based on the scientific literature. It is a well known fact that a diet that lacks sufficient fruits and vegetables (i.e. alkaline or basic foods) has been associated with a risk of osteoporosis.[68] There have been two studies noting the advantage to bones when young girls eat a lot of fruits and vegetables. In the first study, young girls who ate at least 3 servings of fruits and vegetables each day were found to have bigger bones.[69] In another study investigating the effects of fruit intake in girls, concluded that "high intakes of fruit may be important for bone health in girls. It is possible that fruit's alkaline-forming properties mediate the body's acid-base balance." [70] Therefore, next time you eat protein, be good to your bones and eat fruits and/or vegetables at the same time. This will keep your bones healthy, and may reduce the risk of bone disease, such as osteoporosis.

*Calculations based on an average male weight of 80 kg (176 lbs) and an average female weight of 60 kg (136 lbs).

iii) With Protein Comes Fat

A high protein diet is usually accompanied by an increase in dietary fat. Unfortunately, an increase in dietary fat means an increase in the consumption of bad fat (e.g. saturated fat and cholesterol). A diet rich in animal protein, saturated fat, and cholesterol raises low density lipoprotein (LDL), (e.g.

cholesterol) levels. We already know that cholesterol is associated with an increased risk of heart disease. Thereby, eating a diet that is high in protein sources that contain saturated fat and cholesterol is unhealthy. What protein sources are high in saturated fat and cholesterol? Well, hamburgers, steaks, pork, hotdogs, egg yolks, sausages, bacon, lunch meats, cheese, and dairy products are all protein sources that contain saturated fat and cholesterol.

The effect of eating more bad dietary fat causes increases in blood cholesterol levels. This increase in blood cholesterol is compounded in a high-protein/low-carbohydrate diet by the lack of high fibre, high carbohydrate plant foods, such as fruits and vegetables that are known to help lower cholesterol. Therefore, a high protein/low carbohydrate diet is doubly bad for cholesterol levels in the blood. High blood cholesterol levels are a potential negative health effect. This isn't just theoretical. Science has shown that a high protein diet can cause increases in blood cholesterol. A human trial that had subjects use a high-protein diet for 3 months reported that the subjects experienced raised LDL levels.[71] Beware of the fat that may be hiding in the protein you are eating – it can be a problem. Be sure to reach for protein sources that are low in bad fat, such as soy, nuts, fish, chicken and egg whites.

b) The Problem with Fat

Increasing dietary protein can lead to an increase in dietary fat. This increase in animal fat may be a default by North Americans as most accessible sources of protein in our diets are latent in bad fat. Just think of the protein sources at the closest fast food restaurant: burgers, deep fried fish, battered chicken, chili with beef. And, unfortunately, animal fat is generally high in saturated fat and cholesterol - two forms of fat that are known to cause negative health effects in the body, such as heart disease and stroke. In Chapter 5, we'll discuss the various forms of fat and how they work in the body. For now, we simply need to understand that saturated fat and cholesterol are thick, solid-like fats that are hard for our bodies to pump through our small infrastructure of blood vessels.

To date, research on diets high in animal fat (e.g. saturated fat) describes many negative health effects such as heart disease, diabetes and some kinds of cancer. Surprisingly, the first scientific study to truly alarm us about the problems of dietary saturated fat and cholesterol was not published until the 1970s. This first study was large, and thought to be state of the art at its time. It was called The Framingham Study. According to some, the Framingham Study was one of the biggest nutritional awakenings of the 20th century. The study showed that diets high in meat and saturated fat increase the risk for problems such as heart disease, colon cancer, prostate cancer, diabetes, hypertension, osteoporosis, obesity, and decreased lifespan.[72] Let's take a closer look at these associate problems with saturated fat.

i) Fat and Cardiovascular Disease

Fat affects the heart. The fat in our blood affects the health and functionality of our heart and vessels. Eating a lot of saturated fat may increase the number of low density lipoproteins (LDL), the carriers of bad cholesterol in the blood. More LDL means more cholesterol that can be in the blood at one time – a negative biological condition.

A high level of cholesterol in the blood is a major risk factor for heart disease. Elevated levels of LDL in the blood can lead to plaque buildup in the arteries, known as atherosclerosis. Atherosclerosis can start in childhood. These small plaques can form anywhere in the arteries of the body. They are only of concern when they rupture or grow large enough to occlude an artery. As one can guess, when a plaque occludes an artery, the artery cannot let blood pass. If this occlusion is in an artery that supplies blood to the heart muscle, to help the heart pump, the heart will stop. This is a heart attack (i.e. myocardial infarct). If the occluded artery goes to the brain, this is known as a stroke. When a plaque ruptures, it can cause a clotting effect or build up of platelets, just like how a scab form on your skin. This clotting effect is made possible by platelets in the blood that can stick together at a place of injury. Sometimes, these platelets become too effective and can stick together in large numbers and form a clot which can completely block an artery. If this occurs in the brain or in the heart, the result is a heart attack or a stroke.

Atherosclerosis, the formation of plaque on vessel walls, should be a concern to high protein dieters. Human studies have found that a diet rich in animal protein, saturated fat, and cholesterol raises low density lipoprotein (LDL) cholesterol levels (i.e. bad cholesterol)[73], which in turn increases plaque formation. This LDL raising effect is compounded in the high protein/low-carb diet by the lack of high fibre, high carbohydrate plant foods, such as fruits and vegetables that can lower cholesterol. Fruits and vegetables have been scientifically proven to decrease the risk of heart disease.[74,75] Therefore, a diet high in bad fat and low in fruits and vegetables is likely to compromise cardiovascular health.

There are other forms of bad fat that are also affected by a high protein diet. High-fat diets are associated with increasing central obesity. Central or abdominal obesity is known to increase plasma triacylglycerides (i.e. TAGs). Plasma triacylglycerol (TAG) concentration is an important risk factor in relation to the development of cardiovascular disease. Generally, high levels of TAGs are associated with a higher risk of heart disease. How diet, TAGs and heart disease risk are related is unclear. Science appears to contradict itself, likely telling us that we simply do not fully understand the complexity of this interaction. Traditionally, a low-fat, high-carbohydrate diet has been used to reduce bad cholesterol (e.g. LDL) levels. However, such diets can increase TAGs and reduce good cholesterol (e.g. high density lipoprotein). Contrarily, there is strong epidemiological (i.e. population study) evidence that reducing total fat intake is not protective against coronary heart disease.[76] Therefore, it appears to be unclear as to whether a diet low in fat is beneficial to heart health. However, it is consistent in science that a diet high in saturated fat is not healthy for the heart. Science has shown us that saturated fat will increase plasma cholesterol levels, an effect not desirable for heart health.

ii) Fat and Obesity

Perhaps my favorite analogy for the incorrect use of the high-protein/low-carb diet is the idea that low-carb means "buying the hamburger and taking off the top bun". I can get a good laugh from groups on that one. But, all joking aside, there are people who simply don't get the right messages about low carb. Some people do not hear the low carbohydrate message of reducing refined carbohydrates, but the message that it's okay to eat high protein and fat.

Creators of high-protein diets argue that choosing a diet that is high in fat is good for the body. They argue that fat slows the absorption of glucose into the blood stream thereby reducing the gycemic load. This may be correct, however glucose is not the only form of energy. Fat contains a lot of calories (i.e. energy). In fact, fat contains more energy or calories than sugar per gram.

Eating a diet high in fat is not good for your health as we have just seen in the previous section about fat and heart disease. So, how does dietary fat effect your body weight? Well, since fat is the most energy dense form of food in our diet, a diet high in fat may not work out to being the best way to lose weight or maintain a healthy body weight. Yes, slowing the absorption of glucose from the gut works in terms of weight loss because it will help you feel full sooner. However, whether you've consumed fewer calories before you feel full is questionable. If it takes you about 10 minutes into a high fat meal to feel full, have you really consumed less calories than in the 20 minutes it took to feel full when eating a low fat meal? The question is how many of you eat your meals in less than 10 minutes? In fact, most North Americans are eating 2 out of 3 meals in the car, standing up, working, but not sitting down and relaxing.

North Americans are known for overindulging. A review of scientific studies investigating the relationship between energy density of foods and food intake in humans confirms our love to over indulge. The studies showed that humans have a weak innate ability to recognize foods with a high energy density and to appropriately down-regulate the bulk of food eaten in order to maintain energy balance (i.e. passive over-consumption). In other words, we can kind of tell when we are eating high calorie foods, but we are not very good at reducing the total consumption to balance for the higher number of calories we're eating. So, if we were offered a burger and a large salad we are unlikely to be able to recognize that half way through the burger we will have eaten the same amount of energy that there was in the salad.

Most fast foods have an extremely high energy density. On average, North American fast foods have about 65% higher density than the average British diet, more than twice the energy density of recommended healthy diets and, 145% higher than traditional African diets. Therefore, if an African diet represents a diet closest to what our bodies may have evolved from then we are eating 145% more energy than we need each time we pull up to the drive-thru window at our favorite fast food restaurant. The high energy densities of many fast foods challenges human appetite control systems and therefore likely resulting in the accidental consumption of excess energy causing weight gain and obesity.[77] Therefore, perhaps eating the hamburger without the bun may not really be the best way to try to lose weight. It's about the amount of energy or calories that we eat.

When it comes to discussing obesity and fat consumption there are many factors that should be mentioned, not all of which we have considered. Perhaps most important is to clarify that the amount of fat consumed is not directly association with obesity. There are many other factors involved in obesity including overall caloric intake, activity level and genetics.

iii) Fat and Diabetes

Obesity, diet and diabetes are all related. The amount of fat we eat can affect our risk of diabetes. Based on the available evidence on diet and lifestyle in the prevention of type 2 diabetes, it is recommended that a normal weight status (i.e. BMI 21-23) and regular physical activity be maintained throughout adulthood.[78]

Preventing abdominal obesity is also noted as an important way to reduce the risk of diabetes by experts. In other words, obesity is best avoided in the prevention of diabetes.

Experts also note that saturated fat intake should be less than 7% of the total energy intake for the prevention of diabetes.[79] It is well known that a diet high in saturated fat should be avoided as it may be associated with an increased risk of diabetes.[80] It is important that dieters who are diabetics realize that a diet high in saturated fat is not recommended. As well, healthy dieters should be aware that a diet high in saturated fat is not advisable if interested in reducing one's risk of diabetes. The anti-carb, high saturated fat diet that some low-carbohydrate dieters have fallen into, may increase the risk of developing diabetes.

iv) Fat and Cancer

Whether dietary fat intake is directly associated with cancer risk is a large debate. To date there is no overwhelmingly conclusive research on the topic. For example, several studies have suggested that a high intake of fats and fat-rich foods may increase the risk of ovarian cancer. However, the very large Nurses' Health Study cohort of over 80,000 women failed to support this theory.[81] Environmental factors such as lifestyle, pollution, and genetics play a role in the risk of cancer, causing great difficulty in associating fat, or any other one factor with cancer risk.[82]

However, when examining the sum total of the research, some fat subtypes, (saturated fat) and lifestyle changes (obesity, physical activity) may affect the risk and progression of cancers. For example, the European Prospective Investigation of Cancer and

Nutrition (EPIC) Norfolk study involving over 13,000 women between 1993 and 1997 concluded that there was an association between fat, particularly saturated fat, and cancer risk. And, it is well known that high dietary intake of fatty foods is associated with an increased risk of colon cancer.[83] This is enough to raise concern and to send a warning that high fat diets may increase the risk of some types of cancer.

This concern has been raised by government officials. The United Kingdom Food Standards Agency website noted that high-fat, low-carbohydrate diets may increase the risk of cancer and heart disease. With a recent estimate that 3 million people in the United Kingdom are trying low-carbohydrate diets there is growing concern over the potential for such diets to increase the risk of cancer. To date, there is no current evidence linking the Atkin's version of a low-carb diet directly to cancer, diabetes or heart disease.

c) The Problem with No Carbs

The body needs glucose to work. It's our fuel. The body will use glucose (sugar) in the blood as its primary source of energy. Glucose in the blood normally comes from food, primarily carbohydrates, in the gut. Once the blood is depleted of glucose, the body then uses glycogen stores. Glycogen stores are like the battery cells of our muscles. When carbohydrates are lacking in the diet for an extended period of time, the stores become drained. The result of glycogen loss is early fatigue during exercise.[84] If carbohydrates are still not in the diet, and glycogen stores are dry, the body converts to another form of metabolism, called ketosis, to create the needed energy molecules.

Ketosis is a process in which fat is mobilized for metabolism in the body. The idea of breaking down your fat stores for energy may sound great; however, this form of metabolism is not meant to be the everyday way for your body to work. In fact, it's meant to be a way to survive starvation. And, if used for extended periods of time, ketosis may have negative health effects such as elevated levels of non-essential fats in the blood stream, kidney stones, dehydration, and osteoporosis. The elevated levels of bad fats in the blood is caused by the mobilization of fat into the blood stream as it goes from our fat stores to the cells that need them for energy. The resulting kidney stones may be caused by two problems. Firstly, eating a lot of protein causes an excess need for filtration of impurities from the blood by the kidneys. Secondly, the lack of water normally created from carbohydrate metabolism caused dehydration which further challenges the kidneys. Lastly, the potential for developing osteoporosis is caused by the use of calcium from the bones to balance the acidic blood pH resulting from the acidic reactions of ketosis.

Unfortunately, it is not only theory that suggests the low carbohydrate diet may be detrimental to your health. In fact, population studies indicate that the low-carbohydrate diet does cause negative effects on the body. In a study reported by the Physicians Committee for Responsible Medicine that investigated the effects of low-carb diets, 42% of individuals experienced a loss of energy, 22% reduced kidney function, stone or severe infection and 20% heart problems or elevated cholesterol.[85] This is a large percentage of people reporting severe side effects of a low-carbohydrate diet.

Mood is also affected from a lack of carbohydrates. A diet that lacks carbohydrates stops the brain from regulating serotonin, a chemical in the brain that elevates mood and suppresses appetite.[86] This may explain why some people still feel hungry after a high protein meal, like a large steak, despite sufficient caloric intake. Their stomachs are full but their brain doesn't have a quick increase in glucose to cause serotonin production to tell you to stop eating. More importantly, lower levels of serotonin can make you feel irritable and depressed. Many anti-depressant drugs work to increase serotonin levels. Carbohydrates are the feel good food. It's important to eat carbohydrates to maintain a good mood.

Conclusively, we know that our kidneys, bones, brains and energy levels are all affected by the carbohydrates in our diets. In an extensive review of the scientific literature titled, "Low-carbohydrate diets: what are the potential short and long-term health implications?" in *Clinical Nutrition* by Bilsborough and Crowe, the Australian authors state, "Complications such as heart arrhythmias, cardiac contractile function impairment, sudden death, osteoporosis, kidney damage, increased cancer risk, impairment of physical activity and lipid abnormalities can all be linked to long-term restriction of carbohydrates in the diet." The report also noted that short-term hazards of following a high-fat, low-carb diet include impotence and cardiac arrest. This is hypothesized to be due to electrolyte depletion caused by dehydration.[87] This report and the other points noted above paint a poor picture of negative health effects associated with a diet low in carbohydrates.

d) Low-Carb Diets in Those with Dietary Concerns

The use of a high-protein/low-carbohydrate diet has raised concerns about its potential negative biological effects. If these negative biological effects are of concern to the average, healthy North American it raises even greater concern as to the effect of these diets in people with special diets, conditions and diseases.

i) Low-Carb Diets and Diabetes

Blood sugar (i.e. blood glucose) is very important to diabetics as this disease renders them unable to handle their blood sugar effectively. A diabetic does not control their blood sugar well due to the inability of their body to create insulin, or the inability of the body's cells to recognize insulin and to react to it. This represents Type I and Type II diabetes respectively. The overall result is that when sugar reaches the blood stream it is left there – the cells are not able to properly pull it out of the blood and into the cell to use for energy. This means that the blood can have high levels of sugar in it. This is damaging to blood vessels. Long term damage from high blood sugar levels can lead to damage of the small vessels of the eyes, feet and fingers. This is why diabetics are warned about the loss of feeling in their fingers and toes, and retina problems. Therefore, the effect of the foods eaten on the blood sugar level is of particular interest to diabetics.

It's interesting that carbohydrates can influence metabolism by four mechanisms: the type of carbohydrate absorbed, the amount consumed, the rate of absorption and colonic fermentation. The most interesting fact about carbohydrates is that it is not the amount of carbohydrate that improves the body's ability to control blood sugar, but the type of carbohydrate. Wolever, a scientist who studies carbohydrate metabolism, found that reducing carbohydrate intake increases post meal levels of fat in the blood (i.e. post prandial serum fatty-acids) and does not improve overall control of blood sugar in diabetic subjects.[88] In other words, a diet lacking carbohydrates does not improve a diabetic's ability to control glucose. A diet that uses good carbohydrates does. If we refer back to Figure 3, we note that good carbohydrates do not cause the blood sugar level to rise as high, and therefore reduce the damage that carbohydrates can cause to diabetics. Therefore, diabetics should be cautioned from low-carbohydrate diets and the advice of a professional medical practitioner should be sought to determine a diet that best suits individual needs.

Low glycemic diets (i.e. good carbohydrate diets) have been shown in scientific studies to be useful for diabetics. Brand-Miller et al. 2003, preformed a meta-analysis (i.e. review of all scientific studies) of randomized controlled trials to determine whether low-glycemic diets when compared with conventional or high-glycemic diets improved overall blood sugar control in diabetics. They found that choosing a diet with a low glycemic index does improve medium-term markers of blood sugar control.[89] Therefore, a diet that includes low glycemic index foods, or good carbohydrates, may be beneficial to diabetics.

Diabetics also have concern with fatty acid levels in their blood. Low glycemic foods, such as good carbohydrates, are associated with higher good cholesterol levels (HDL) and lower triglyceride levels.[90] Therefore, it appears that good carbohydrates in the diet are beneficial to diabetics to help them control their blood sugar and to improve the fats in their blood as well.

ii) Low-Carb Diets and Pregnancy

One of the greatest concerns with the anti-carbohydrate phenomenon is the lack of some essential nutrients in the diet. This is clearly a problem as even Dr. Atkin's recommends that his high-protein/low-carb diet includes a daily multi-vitamin and mineral. One nutrient in particular that is being missed in low-carbohydrate diets is folate. Folate is added to most carbohydrate foods as it is needed to prevent neuronal tube defects, such as spina bifida, in infants.

Folate is a water-soluble B vitamin. It is normally found in green vegetables, like celery and spinach. However, the lack of fruit and vegetable consumption by North Americans has left our society generally deficient in this nutrient. To prevent an epidemic of neural tube birth defects, both the Canadian and United States government have required that breads, grain products and cereals are fortified with folate. The recommended daily amount of folate for women of childbearing age is 400 micrograms per day.[91] However, the anti-carbohydrate diet trend means that many North Americans are not consuming folate in sufficient amounts and may be increasing the risk of birth defects.
The anti-carbohydrate trend is not only dangerous to women of childbearing age. Dietary folate intake is inversely associated with the risk of colorectal cancer.[92] Colorectal cancer is the second leading cause of cancer-related death in the United States.[93]

Also, B vitamins are involved in the metabolism of homocysteine. Homocysteine is a type of fat found in blood vessels. A high level of homocysteine in the blood is thought to be a potential risk factor for heart disease. Homocysteine is thought to be involved in the disease, atherosclerosis, which causes the hardening of blood vessels and can lead to heart attacks and strokes. As vitamin B is needed in the body to convert homocystiene into less a harmful compound, a diet low or deficient in B vitamins appears to have negative health effects on the heart.

Another concern for women of child bearing age is that a moderately high protein diet could reduce a woman's chance of becoming pregnant. Research from the *European Society of*

Human Reproduction and Embryology in 2004 noted that a diet containing 25% protein disrupted the normal genetic imprinting pattern of mice embryos and adversely affected embryo implantation.[94] In other words, a diet higher in protein than the current national average caused a decreased rate of embryo implantation in mice, and therefore fewer pregnancies. Of note, there was no indication to the amount of carbohydrates consumed in the study. However, low-carb diets tend to be high in protein and therefore, woman trying to conceive should use caution when considering high protein diets. Advice of a qualified medical practitioner should be sought.

Also, what about the effects of a high protein diet on the heart health of a fetus? Early in 2003, research done by Dr. Paul Taylor, of St. Thomas' Hospital, London, England, reported that women who ate a high fat diet during pregnancy may be increasing the risk that their child will develop heart problems in later life.[95] Therefore, a diet high in animal fat, such as most high protein diets, appears to compromise fetal heart health.

To ensure a diet contains sufficient folate, multi-vitamins, fortified grain products and green foods (e.g. green plants, algae and cereal grasses) might be considered. A healthy low-carbohydrate diet should contain good carbohydrates (i.e. complex carbohydrates, or whole wheat) and plenty of vegetables which are necessary to ensure health. Pregnant women should always consult a qualified medical practitioner to discuss their dietary needs.

iii) Low-Carb Diets and Vegetarians:

How does the high protein/low-carbohydrate diet fit into a vegetarian ideal? Vegetarians also need to be aware of what type of carbohydrate they are ingesting. For example, vegetarians may pick up a granola bar at the check out line and not realize that it is full of refined sugar. This granola bar has a high glycemic index and should therefore be avoided if you are on a high protein/low carbohydrate diet. A low-carb vegetarian diet should focus on vegetable sources of protein, such as soy foods, lentils, nuts, nut butters, flaxseeds, sunflower and sesame seeds and tofu. It is possible for vegetarians to do a low-carbohydrate diet. You simply need to remember that fruits and particularly vegetables are sources of "good" carbohydrates and they need not be eliminated from a low-carb diet.[96]

iv) Carbs and Athletes

Athletes are always concerned about fueling their bodies effectively. However, some are tempted by the promises of weight loss from high protein/low-carbohydrate diets. As noted before, carbohydrates are our fuel. Running your body, (e.g. swimming, biking, and dancing) without carbohydrates is like trying to run your car without gas. Muscles contain battery cells called glycogen cells. These provide energy to the muscle during exercise. These battery cells are full of carbohydrate derived fuel. When the diet lacks carbohydrates the body uses glycogen cell energy. This leaves little energy in the battery cells of our muscles when physical activity begins. As you can imagine that means that your muscles contain battery cells that are half drained and therefore cannot perform optimally. The result of a diet lacking sufficient carbohydrates is quick fatigue of the muscles in exercise and poor athletic performance. Therefore, a diet lacking in carbohydrates is not ideal for athletes.

85

Researchers have noted that after a workout the body craves carbohydrates as it seeks to refill the glycogen cells. Japanese researchers from the University of Health and Sport Sciences in Osaka noted in a 2004 study that intake of carbohydrate-rich goods just after exercise is crucial for the body's recovery. However, they also noted that the body does not prefer sweet carbohydrates, such as sucrose.[97] Therefore, the body is naturally craving high quality carbohydrates, re-enforcing the concept that a healthy diet is one that does contain carbohydrates, particularly the good carbohydrates. Also, athletes should be reaching for high quality carbohydrates after a workout, despite the current theory that a large protein meal is required. Don't forget the carbs!

Guidelines for the training diet of athletes were proposed by a group of researchers after they reviewed the scientific literature on post-exercise glycogen storage. It is common knowledge that athletes should ensure they consume enough carbohydrates to meet the fuel requirements of their training programs and to optimize the re-fueling of muscle glycogen cells between workouts.[98] Researchers are discovering that the types of food needed to optimize the energy stored in muscles may be different based on the type of athletic event preformed. The choice of diet for optimal physical performance depends on several factors, including type and duration of exercise, total energy expenditure, time for recovery, dietary preference of the athlete, and whether or not the sporting event is unassisted (and hence athletes are required to transport their food). [99]

For all athletes, carbohydrate-rich foods with a moderate to high glycemic index should be the major carbohydrate choices in recovery meals as they provide a readily available source of carbohydrate for muscle glycogen synthesis. Endurance athletes are particularly encouraged by researchers to ingest a high carbohydrate diet prior to competition to maximize the availability of muscle glycogen. However, in unassisted events there is some thought that a diet higher in fat may be more beneficial.[100] Researchers are currently investigating the importance of triglycerides, a type of fat, in muscle performance.[101] However, to date there is no evidence that diets which are high in fat and restricted in carbohydrate enhance training.

Another concern with the use of low carbohydrate diets by athletes is the effect of carbohydrate restriction on body composition. Restrictions on carbohydrate consumption can result in the loss of lean muscle tissue.[102] Yet, for years we've been hearing how wonderful lean muscle tissue is as it burns more calories than other forms of muscle. For the past decade we've strived to increase our lean muscle mass, yet now we're using a diet that causes us to lose this valuable tissue type. In addition, lean muscle tissue can give the body an appearance of fitness and tone - a much desired look of this century.

Hence, a low-carbohydrate diet appears to go against some current theories on muscle and athletic health. Athletes should be sure that their diets are not lacking in carbohydrates to guarantee proper muscle performance.

v) Carbs and Disease

Many low-carb advocates will argue that there are many studies denoting that diets high in carbohydrates are associated with disease. We've just discussed the issue of diabetes, a common rebuttal from low-carb advocates to the importance in lowering carbohydrate intake in the diet of diabetics. However, as noted, it is not the total carbohydrates that matter, but the type of carbohydrate.

Another example is a study noted by the *Journal of Cancer Epidemiology Biomarkers in Prevention*. In this study, they compared 475 women who had been recently diagnosed with breast cancer to a control group of women who did not have the disease. They found the women who had breast cancer eat more simple carbohydrates than the controls. They also noted that diets higher in insoluble fibre (e.g. complex carbohydrates) had a lower risk of breast cancer.[103] In other words, eating the good carbohydrates is beneficial to health. Eating bad carbohydrates, (i.e. the simple carbohydrates) that are full of sucrose and fructose, can be detrimental to your body and may be associated with an increased risk of disease.

Therefore, when arguments are made against carbohydrate consumption because studies associate them with an increased risk of disease, one must evaluate which type of carbohydrate it is. Science shows that good carbohydrates are beneficial to health, and that some diseases can be caused or related to a lack of carbohydrates in the diet.

Chapter 5:
The Facts on Fat

Fat. The world is tainted. It's almost as bad as those naughty four letter words we use in times of frustration. When we hear the word fat, we all seem to feel a little shutter go through our bodies. We all think, "Am I?" We live in a fat phobic society. This 'fat phobia' has been created over a number of years. Our fat phobia is founded on four key elements: historical obsession with diets, media coverage, the 'Barbie Phenomenon' that thin is desirable and, scientific association between fat intake and chronic diseases, such as cancer and heart disease.

The last two decades of our fat obsession has left its marks. Store aisles are full of low fat, fat-free labels. North Americans have tried for the past decade to eat less fat. However, even though we're eating less fat, we've gotten fatter. The percentage of overweight Americans has jumped from 55.9% to 64.5% in the last decade.[104] Why? 1) We eat too much and exercise too little. 2) Weight loss is not just about fat consumption. 3) Some fats are harmful.

There are many fallacies and phobias about fat. Let's focus on the two most important. Firstly, being fat is not necessarily due to the consumption of fat. Obesity is not directly related to eating fat. And, secondly, not all fat is created equally. There are many types of fat, each with its own pros and cons. So, let's get the facts on fat.

a) Obesity

According to the *International Obesity Task Force (IOTF)*, in 2003 there were 1.7 billion obese people worldwide.[105] In fact, the statistics on obesity are staggering.

- 1.1 billion people are overweight or obese.
  (Source: IOTF, 2003)

- 1.7 billion are at risk of a range of weight-related illnesses which include type 2 diabetes, heart disease and some common cancers. *(Source: IOTF,. 2003)*

- *The International Diabetes Federation* estimates that there are 190 million people with diabetes and this is forecast to increase to 330 million by 2025.

- United States – 16% of children are obese*

- United States – childhood obesity is most prevalent in African-American and Latino girls*

- United States - more than 64% of adults are either over-weight or obese. *(*Source: 1999-2000 National Health and Nutrition Examination Survey (NHANES))*

- Ontario, Canada - Almost one of every 2 adults are obese or overweight.

- Canada – 48% of adults are overweight, 15% are obese.
  (Source: Statistics Canada, 2002)

- United Kingdom – obesity rates have doubled since the 1980s. *(Source: United Kingdom Department of Health, Trend Data for Adults 1993-2000)*

- United Kingdom - 5.5% of boys and 7.2% of girls, aged 2-15 years, are obese *(Source: Health Survey for England, 2002)*

- European Union – 24% of children are overweight. *(Source: IOTF, 2002)*

This is a great concern as obesity is linked with many diseases, including diabetes, heart disease, and cancer, such as endometrial cancer, a condition that affects the lining of the uterus.[106] Being fat is linked with being ill. What is causing us to be so fat?

Did you know that one pound of fat represents about 3,500 excess calories? Since the body cannot store excess protein or carbohydrates, it converts them into fat for storage. Therefore, the consumption of fat does not directly relate to the obesity of a person. The amount of fat on your body is not directly related to the amount of fat you consume. So, don't blame fat for being fat.

What causes obesity? Is obesity caused by having a slower metabolism? A meta-analysis (i.e. a review of all the scientific papers) on energy expenditure in obese people concluded that the cause of obesity is "far from certain". Some like to believe that obesity is caused by a slow metabolism. However, it has not yet been scientifically proven that obesity is caused by a slow metabolism.[107] In fact, it is not likely to be the sole cause of this epidemic. Therefore, if slow metabolism is not the cause then what is making us so fat?

Despite the increasing prevalence of obesity, there is no evidence to support the view that obesity is caused by increased intake of fat. Obesity has more to do with the number of calories you

91

consume. Foods that have a lot of calories in them, also known as calorie-dense foods, include those that are high in fat. Despite the lack of association between obesity and increased fat intake, one need remember that fat is a calorie-dense foods which may cause obesity.

Are we obese because of our consumption of calorie-rich foods? Big portions, such as the 'Biggie Sized' meal options at fast food restaurants, encourage people to eat more. In fact, a recent trip I took noted the North American love to-up size our foods. This was one of my notorious road trips when there were a lot of kilometers covered in a short period of time. On this trip, I bought a medium tea in Ontario at a popular coffee shop in the morning. Then, just after noon I was in New York State, and ordered a medium again at the same popular coffee shop. To my surprise, the cup was a full size larger than the one I had in the morning. A medium in New York was a large in Ontario. We love to increase the sizes of our food portions. This is not the only example. North American proportions are always being compared. Did you know that in the 1950s the standard serving size for a soda was 12 ounces? Today it's 24 ounces. In fact, a serving has grown a lot, as at one chain of convenience stores they serve a cup of soda that is the equivalent of a half galloon, and call it a serving.

Is this healthy? Does it affect out calorie consumption? Studies have found that big portions of calorie dense foods may boost calorie consumption even higher without providing any additional satisfaction.[108] In other words, eating the biggie sized fries causes us to eat more calories as there are more fries to eat, but it doesn't provide us with a proportionally increased feeling of satisfaction in our stomach from eating that much more. Calorie density and portion size add together to affect caloric intake. Since, caloric intake is known to be associated with weight management, the combination of biggie sized calorie dense food is a real obesity problem. Thereby, biggie sizes of calorie dense foods are making our fight against weight management more difficult. Scientists have confirmed that eating too much calorie-rich food can lead to obesity. [109]

Yet, we know that a biggie size fries is not the best for us, and we still consume it. Why? According to some scientists, eating calorie-rich food seems to calm the nerves, which may explain why such foods have become an entrenched part of our stressed-out North American lifestyles. This is a grave problem as science has found that eating too much calorie-rich food can lead to depression and more stress. [110]

In a Harvard journal article on our eating habits, author Craig Lambert states that "30 percent of American children aged four to 19 eat fast food, and older and wealthier ones eat even more. Overall, 7 percent of the U.S. population visits McDonald's each day, and 20 to 25 percent eat in some kind of fast-food restaurant." [111] In Japan cars are not sold with cup holders – perhaps a sign of fast foods influence on our North American lifestyles. In fact, the size of cup holders in the North American versions of cars have been increasing in size over the past decade to accommodate the ever growing biggie sized soft drinks at our favorite fast food drive-thrus. There is a serious problem not only with our food choices, but with the way our lifestyles are accommodating and accepting the fast food, calorie-dense, biggie sized way of life.

All in all, according to science, the best option for the prevention of obesity and cardiovascular disease is a modest reduction in fat intake to 30-35% of the total energy consumed, with the bulk of carbohydrates being derived from complex carbohydrates.[112]How do we get there? First, we learn more about fat and how there are different types. There is both good and bad fat.

b) Types of Fat

There are many types of fat. More than I could ever explain. However, the important thing to know is that some fats are worse than others. The worst fat is trans fat. Trans fatty acids are found in processed foods like margarine. A few years back as the fear of saturated fat emerged, the food industry switched from using butter in processed foods to using vegetable oil. This reduced the amount of saturated fat and cholesterol, appealing the fat phobia of the time. The food industry had to partially hydrogenate the vegetable oil to make it stable in heat. During the process of hydrogenation, trans fats are formed. This manufacturing solution to the desire of the public to reduce the amount of saturated fat in a product unleashed the creation of an even more concerning fat – trans fat.

Trans fatty acids are present in food items like crackers, cookies, French fries, hot chocolate mixes, some cereals, and foods with ingredients such as partially hydrogenated vegetable oil and shortening. If the amount of trans fats is not present in the nutritional facts panel, simply add up the value of the saturated, polyunsaturated and monounsaturated fats and subtract that from the total fat. The amount remaining is the amount of trans fats in the product. Of note, margarine can also be source of trans fatty acids. The main message is to read the label carefully. Why are trans fats to bad? Well, trans fats are like Mack trucks on the freeway. They are big, slow and can block the flow of traffic.

In your blood stream, trans fats are like Mack trucks on your freeway, known as your blood vessels. Also, trans fats are not a normal substance for the body to metabolize. The body does not need trans fats for any structures or functions. It's just big, useless and gets in the way. Metabolic studies have shown that *trans* fats have adverse effects on blood lipid levels—increasing LDL ("bad") cholesterol while decreasing HDL ("good") cholesterol. This combined effect on the ratio of LDL to HDL cholesterol is double that of saturated fatty acids.[113] Trans fats have also been associated with an increased risk of coronary heart disease in epidemiologic studies.[114] Also, in 1994, a group of scientist from Harvard used metabolic studies to estimate that approximately 30,000 premature coronary heart disease deaths annually could be attributable to consumption of trans fatty acids.[115] Avoiding trans fats is part of a healthy diet. A longer discussion on trans fats will follow.

Saturated fats are typically solid at room temperatures. Saturated fats include cholesterol; the number one monitored risk factor for heart disease in North America of the past decade. Saturated fats can be found in meats, dairy products, butter and most processed foods. Saturated fats lower good cholesterol (HDL) and raise bad cholesterol (LDL) levels, thereby increasing the risk of cardiovascular disease.[116] Saturated fats should be consumed at a minimum in your daily diet. Why not recommend avoiding saturated fat? Saturated fat includes cholesterol which is a key component of many aspects of the human body. The liver can manufacture cholesterol as it is an important element required in cell membranes. This is why you may have heard the expression that even if you do not eat fat you will still have it in your body. For many North Americans who suffer from high cholesterol

95

levels eliminating dietary cholesterol may not result in lower blood cholesterol levels as in some people it is an over production of cholesterol by the liver, an enzyme called HMG-CoA, that causes their elevated levels.

Monounsaturated fats are typically liquid at room temperature and are easily seen on food labels across North America. These fats are not of great concern. The Mediterranean diet, which gets rave reviews for its healthy effects, is a diet that is high in monounsaturated fatty acids. In fact, a diet high in monounsaturated fatty acids may have healthy benefits for the heart and memory. Monounsaturates are found in plant oils like corn, safflower and canola oil.

Polyunsaturated fatty acids are the best fats of all. Polyunsaturated fatty acids are a large group of fats that include the essential fatty acids (e.g. linoleic acid (LA) and alpha linolenic acid (LNA)). Generically, some people refer to essential fatty acids as omega-3, omega-6 and omega-9 as these are the families of polyunsaturated fats that LA and LNA belong too. Essential fatty acids (EFAs) are called essential because your body cannot manufacture them – you must consume them to have them in your body. For this reason, many North Americans are deficient in these healthy fats as fish and flax are not a large part of our diets.

EFAs are required for the proper functioning and structure of every cell in the body, and therefore are critical for optimal health. EFAs increase the absorption of vitamins and minerals; promote proper nerve functioning; help produce hormones; nourish the skin, hair and nails; ensure normal growth and development; and help prevent and likely treat disease. Deficiency of EFAs has been shown in many scientific studies to result in a wide array of symptoms. These include skin problems, cell death, loss of visual acuity, fatigue, neuropathies, impaired growth and fertility, failure to thrive, organ damage and increased occurrence of illness and death. One can see how this might happen when we look at the number of cell processes that EFAs influence: regulation of enzymes, gene expression, and cell signaling pathways, gene activation, receptor function and activation, membrane permeability, attachment of proteins to fatty acids, oxidation of fats, cell communication with nucleus, lipid signaling and transport systems.

EFAs are a vital part of cell membranes. You are what you eat. If you eat butter, which is hard at room temperature, your cell membranes are also hard. On the other hand, if you eat polyunsaturated fatty acids, including essential fatty acids your cell membranes are more fluid which improves other physical properties and structural functions of the cell. A fluid cell membrane allows the cell to transport signals and nutrients more effectively and efficiently. Just imagine how difficult it would be to increase and decrease the width of your blood vessels if your cells were not fluid. Every time you changed your hydration level, change your heart rate or blood pressure your vessels would not be able to adjust to keep the system working.

The EFAs, LA and LNA fit into two families. LNA is an omega 3 fatty acid. LA is an omega 6 fatty acid. Each of which has its own story to tell about how they improve the body's ability to function.

Omega-3 fatty acids are found in fish, flax and, to a limited extent, hemp. The body loves ALA. It will use D6D, an enzyme that is in high demand in the body, to break down LNA into eicosapentaenoic acid (EPA) and docosahexaenoic acid (DHA) before it breaks down other fats, such as omega-6s. Fatty acids have many roles in improving cell functions and structures. Perhaps the most important role is the production of hormones that can affect the overall health of the body. EPA is converted in the body to a number of various hormones that can dilate and constrict blood vessels, and mildly decrease inflammation and inhibit blood clotting. EPA hormones are most useful as defense mechanisms against trauma and infection. DHA has a more important role than hormones. DHA is a vital component of the nerves, eyes and brain.

Linoleic acid (LA) is an omega-6 fatty acid. LA is generally found in plant oils such as borage oil, evening primrose oil, hemp oil and more. In the body, LA is converted by the D6D enzyme into gamma linolenic acid (GLA). Then, GLA can be converted in the body into a hormone called PGE1. This hormone reduces inflammation, increases vessel dilation and inhibits blood clotting. As one can see these are affects that are very helpful in reducing disease. In fact, science has found omega-6 fatty acids to be beneficial for cardiovascular, skin and joint health.[117,118] As inflammation is a key part of many diseases, it is likely that we will soon learn of other diseases that GLA can help prevent and perhaps treat. Of note, it is not the LA, the essential fat that is so important to our health, but the GLA that it is converted into. In the typical North American diet we consume a ratio of about 40:1 of omega-6 to omega-3. Therefore, some people think that omega-6 is not healthy as a supplement. However, it is important to know that the omega-6 noted in the above ratio is mostly LA, not GLA. Since we can see that GLA has many direct healthy benefits that can help prevent and treat many common day illnesses, it is vital that we supplement with a good source of GLA, such as borage oil and evening primrose oil.

Why is it important to supplement with GLA? Good fat can be good for nothing if your D6D enzyme is not working effectively. The following conditions can impair the ability of the D6D enzyme to convert LA to GLA, and LNA to EPA and DHA.

a. high intake of saturated fats
b. high intake of LA (refined oils such as canola, sunflower, safflower and corn oils)
c. smoking
d. alcohol consumption
e. stress
f. ageing
g. premature infants (D6D is not effective until 6 months)
h. viral infection
i. diabetes
j. cancer

Therefore, it is vital that North Americans consume through diet or supplementation proper amounts of EPA, DHA and GLA as these good fats play an important role in our health management and maintenance.

As one can see omega fatty acids are very important in the proper functioning of the body. Therefore, it is not surprising that scientists have found some associations between omega fatty acids and chronic diseases such as Alzheimer's, depression, heart disease, arthritis, and cancer.[119]

Proper utilization of fats by the body depends on a proper ratio of good and bad fats. Our ratio of 40:1 should really be 4:1. To do this we need to eat less refined oils and saturated fat, supplement with good fats and eat fish and flax more often.

What about omega-9? Omega-9s are part of a good fatty acid supplementation regime as they help ensure that a healthy balance of good fats is obtained, even though they aren't essential. Generally, omega-9 fatty acids are present in all plant oils. And, recently science is discovering that omega-9 fatty acid may also play a key role in a healthy body. Recent research found that oleic acid, an omega-9 fatty acid help fight against breast cancer as it negatively affects a common gene receptor.[120] Oleic acid is the chief fatty acid in olive oil.

Later in this chapter we'll discuss more about the science of essential fatty acids.

DIETARY FATS			
Type of Fat	Main Source	State at Room Temperature	Effect on Cholesterol Levels
Monounsaturated	Olives; olive oil, canola oil, peanut oil; cashews, almonds, peanuts, and most other nuts; avocados	Liquid	Lowers LDL; raises HDL
Polyunsaturated	Corn, soybean, safflower, and cottonseed oils; fish	Liquid	Lowers LDL; raises HDL
Saturated	Whole milk, butter, cheese, and ice cream; red meat; chocolate; coconuts, coconut milk, and coconut oil	Solid	Raises both LDL and HDL
Trans	Most margarines; vegetable shortening; partially hydrogenated vegetable oil; deep-fried chips; many fast foods; most commercial baked goods	Solid or semi-solid	Raises LDL

Percentage of Specific Types of Fat in Common Oils and Fats*				
Oils	Saturated	Mono-unsaturated	Poly-unsaturated	Trans
Canola	7	58	29	0
Safflower	9	12	74	0
Sunflower	10	20	66	0
Corn	13	24	60	0
Olive	13	72	8	0
Soybean	16	44	37	0
Peanut	17	49	32	0
Palm	50	37	10	0
Coconut	87	6	2	0
Cooking Fats				
Shortening	22	29	29	18
Lard	39	44	11	1
Butter	60	26	5	5
Margarine/Spreads				
70% Soybean Oil, Stick	18	2	29	23
67% Corn & Soybean Oil Spread, Tub	16	27	44	11
48% Soybean Oil Spread, Tub	17	24	49	8
60% Sunflower, Soybean, and Canola Oil Spread, Tub	18	22	54	5

*Values expressed as percent of total fat; data are from analyses at Harvard School of Public Health Lipid Laboratory and U.S.D.A. publications.

c) The Trouble with Trans Fat

We are eating a lot of trans fat. To explain, according to experts, the total fat and saturated fat intakes, as a percentage of total energy, has been declining over the past 30 years in the United States.[121] This is positive news. However, the majority of individuals, regardless of age, reported consuming a diet that is greater than the recommended levels of fat and saturated fatty acids by the Dietary Guidelines for Americans. Total fat intake has not decreased as greatly as saturated fat intake. Therefore, we're eating more of another fat. Dietary patterns show us that due to thoughts that foods with less saturated fat are healthier, we are eating more trans fat than before. In fact, some news reports suggest some of us are eating up to 20g of trans fat per day.

What's so scary about trans fatty acids? Well, firstly, they are everywhere. Secondly, they may be harmful. In the 1990s, epidemiological studies discovered that trans fatty acids increase the risk of coronary heart disease.[122] Coronary heart disease involves the formation of fatty plaques on the lining of the inside of blood vessels. The cells that line the inside of blood vessels are called endothelia. Over time plaque builds up on the endothelium. Scientific studies have not confirmed the mechanisms or specific details of how trans fat increase the risk of coronary heart disease. However, the results of in vitro studies have shown that trans fatty acids cause a significant increase in secretion of reactive oxygen species, interleukin-6, tumor necrosis factor alpha and metalloproteinase-9, and enhance apoptosis (i.e. cell death) from endothelium. This causes damage to the endothelium lining the blood vessels. If plaque is over these damaged cells, the plaque can rupture. This causes the body to respond by trying to repair the rupture with platelets –

similar to how a scab forms on your skin when you cut yourself. However, in a blood vessel there is limited room and if the "scab" becomes too big it can block the blood vessel. This is a problem if this is a major artery to the heart or the brain. All in all it appears that trans-fatty acids may destroy blood vessel lining integrity and cause plaque rupture, all accepted markers of enhanced atherosclerosis risk,[123] a cardiovascular disease.

Another health concern of trans fats is that they may impair the metabolism of essential fatty acids in humans. This is most concerning as it can effect the development of babies. Essential fatty acids (e.g. long-chain polyunsaturates) are of great physiological importance during prenatal and postnatal development. They are key elements in the brain, blood, and eyes. Consumption of trans fatty acids during pregnancy may inhibit the mother's body from metabolizing essential fatty acids, thereby reducing the amount available to the fetus for development. Also, during breast feeding, trans fatty acids from a mother's diet end up in breast milk. The amount of trans fatty acids found in human milk vary between countries; 0.35% in Africa to 7.2% in Canada.[124] The negative effects of high levels of trans fats in human milk on breast-fed infants is not yet well documented but are concerning.

The grave health concerns of trans fat have prompted companies to remove trans fatty acids from their products. In fact, the United States will introduce mandatory trans fatty acid labeling in 2006. The Canadian government has similar plans. More interesting, Walmart, the largest retailer in the United States and perhaps soon to be in North America, has made statements that in 2005 they will only sell trans fat free foods.

103

Trans fatty acids may not be fully understood by the scientific community, however, since they do not offer any nutritional value, they may interfere with essential fatty acid metabolism and appear to be damaging to the cardiovascular system. Therefore, trans fats are likely best avoided.

d) Benefits of Omega Fatty Acids

Some of you may know the 3 main classes of polyunsaturated fatty acids as omega-3, omega-6 and omega-9. Many polyunsaturated fatty acids play a key role in disease prevention. Some polyunsaturated fatty acids are essential: LA and LNA. Essential means that they have to be consumed, the body cannot make them. Essential fatty acids are important as they must be consumed in order for the body to have them. Also, because essential fatty acids are converted into other good fats, essential fats are needed for proper fat ratios and health. Science has been discovering that the good fats play a key role in preventing many major North American diseases. The topic of omega fatty acids research could fill an entire book, so let's just do a quick review of the current science on omegas and diseases.

i) Omegas and Cardiovascular Disease

Many know that heart disease is the number one cause of death in North America, killing over a million people each year. However, many do not know that fats can actually help the heart. Omega-3 fatty acids help fight cardiovascular disease by reducing platelet clumping potential, decreasing platelet/vessel wall interactions and altering triglyceride levels. In fact, reviews of the current scientific research suggests that omega-3 fatty acid supplementation appears to work effectively with pharmaceuticals such as lovastatin to lower lipid levels[125] and fish oil may be as effective as pharmaceuticals in improving heart health. More impressively, is omega-3 fatty acids' ability to reduce the risk of sudden death from cardiovascular disease in post myocardial infarct patients. In fact, heart attack patients will be excited to know that omega-3 supplementation can reduce the risk of death from a second heart attack, a very common occurrence, by 45%.[126] Obviously, the research strongly suggests that fish oil or omega-3 fatty acids can help treat and prevent cardiovascular disease. This is reflected in the American Heart Association's recommendations of 900mg/day of omega-3 fatty acids.[127]

ii) Omegas and Arthritis

Omega-3 fatty acids are helpful for arthritis. Arthritis is the inflammation of the joint. As we've already mentioned, omega-3 fatty acids can help with inflammation. A Mediterranean diet, which has as much as 40% of its fat in the form of omega-3s, has been shown to significantly lessen symptoms of rheumatoid arthritis.[128] Therefore, omega-3s in the form of fish or flax are great additions to a joint healthy diet.

Arthritis is typically treated with non-steroidal anti-inflammatory drugs (i.e. NSAIDs). These decrease the inflammation by stopping the action of cyclo-oxygenase, a mediator in the inflammation pathway. However, NSAIDs can have side effects such as ulcers. Of even greater concern is the potential increase in risk of stroke associated with a form of NSAIDs (i.e. a cyclo-oygenase II inhibitor) that prompted the removal of a very popular anti-inflammatory, Vioxx, from the market. Clinical trails show that GLA (gamma linolenic acid), an omega-6 fatty acid, might be able to replace pharmaceutical drugs in the treatment of arthritis.[129] However, GLA does not solve the problem. It appears that GLA supplementation is helpful because GLA is converted into hormones that result in less damaging inflammation than other forms of fat.[130] Even though GLA may not be the solution to arthritis, it has been shown in studies to repair the damage that NSAIDs can cause (e.g. ulcers)[131], and therefore may be part of a healthy arthritis program.

iii) Omega 3s and Attention Deficit and Hyperactive Disorder (ADHD)

Did you know that 20% of the fat in your brain is DHA, an omega-3 fatty acid? Omega-3 fatty acids are vital for neurotransmission and maintenance of normal brain function. It is hypothesized by some that DHA levels in the diet and brain may be somehow associated with behavior problems, like AD(H)D.

Attention Deficit/Hyperactivity Disorder (ADHD) is the most common behavioral disorder in children. ADHD is characterized by attention deficit, impulsivity, and sometimes over-activity ("hyperactivity"). When scientists compared AD(H)D patients with non-hyperactive patients, they found that AD(H)D children were deficient in omega-3 fatty acids, and some where deficient in omega-6 as well.[132] Scientists also reported that children who have AD(H)D have greater biomarkers of DHA oxidation, suggesting a mechanical problem with DHA breakdown.[133]

Clinical supplementation trials have been limited, and have not yet shown a statistically significant improvement in AD(H)D symptoms. However, further research is warranted and is promising. There have been a few trials with significant results using combos of omega-3 and omega-6. Watch scientific journals for future updates on this topic.

iv) Omegas and Cancer

Omega-3 fatty acids may also help with cancer. Research on animals has shown that omega-3 fatty acids can slow the growth of cancer, increase the efficacy of chemotherapy and reduce the side effects of the chemotherapy.[134]

The American Institute for Cancer Research estimates that 30-40% of cancers in the world are preventable by feasible dietary means. Dietary fat can have a positive or a negative effect on breast cancer. It matters what type of fat is consumed. Population studies have linked diets high in saturated fats with an increased risk of breast cancer.

Meanwhile, essential fatty acids are well known for their ability to decrease the risk of cancer. For example, GLA (gamma-linolenic acid), an omega-6 fatty acid, has been shown to kill about 40 different human cancer cell lines in vitro without harming normal cells.[135]

Most commonly, flax, a source of LNA, is thought of as the cancer fighter. Research has linked dietary consumption of flax seeds to an improvement in hormone levels in menopausal women.[136] Perhaps more convincing is research from the University of Toronto which had newly diagnosed breast cancer patients eating two tablespoons of ground flaxseed each day.[137] This small study was the first to suggest that flax components may in fact help fight cancer. Despite limited scientific evidence flax is possibly a role in the prevention of breast cancer.

In general, a diet low in bad fat (i.e. saturated, trans and cholesterol), and high in good fats (i.e. omega fatty acids) may be helpful in the prevention and fight against cancer.

v) Omegas and Pregnancy

A growing body of scientific evidence suggests that fish oil is healthy for moms and for the fetus. In fact, research even suggests that fish oil consumption during pregnancy may be good for the child later in life.

In the October issue of the *Journal of Nutrition*, scientists reported that supplementing with fish oil during pregnancy results in a lower risk of some adult diseases in offspring. They reported that maternal supplementation of fish oil was beneficial in maintaining circulating glucose, insulin, cholesterol and homocysteine levels in the adult offspring.[138] Therefore, it appears that mothers who supplement with fish oil during pregnancy may help their offspring have a better chance of avoiding adult diseases, such as heart disease, stroke and diabetes.

Better yet, fish oil supplementation by mothers may reduce an offspring's chance of developing cancer later in life. A recent scientific study reported that lifelong consumption of a diet rich in n-3 PUFAs, (i.e. omega-3 fatty acids) may protect against tumor growth and cancer.[139] This shows promise that maternal fish oil supplementation may also prevent the development of cancer as adults in their offspring.

These scientific studies showing that fish oil supplementation during pregnancy can have long term effects are not the only good news scientists have announced recently about fish oil.

Research has shown omega-3 fatty acid supplementation has been associated with improved gestation and post-partum depression. Also, researchers from the University of Glasgow reported that DHA supplementation promoted central visual pathway development.[140] This is not surprising as 10-50% of the retina is DHA.

Fetal development also requires arachidonic acid, another important "good" (i.e. polyunsaturated) fat. Arachidonic acid is an omega-6 fatty acid. It is abundant in the diet, as it is found in animal fats. Therefore, it's found in eggs, and in animal and fish fat. Arachidonic acid is a precursor to hormones, that have effects including vascular constriction and pro-inflammation. The transport of arachidonic acid from the mother's blood across the placenta to the baby is of critical importance to fetal growth and development.[141] As more than 90% of a baby's fat is deposited in the last 10 weeks of pregnancy its not surprising that studies suggest that premature babies may be more prone to central nervous system injuries.[142] Therefore, remember arachidonic acid when thinking about good fats for a healthy pregnancy.

Therefore, a diet rich in omega fatty acids appears to be a healthy diet for moms and babies. Maternal fish oil supplementation appears to help with lengthening gestation, reducing post-partum depression, improve fetal eye development and reduce the risk of later life diseases. What a great gift for a fetus – fish oil for short term and long term health.

vi) Omegas and Weight Loss

Imagine eating fat to lose fat. It's not that easy but some science suggests that eating a particular type of fat may assist weight loss if used in a proper weight loss plan that includes a restricted diet and exercise. Conjugated linoleic acid (CLA) is a good fat that has been shown in some scientific studies to help with weight loss. It is not a magical pill. However, it does show some promise in encouraging processes that are favorable for weight loss. One notable study, of decent sample size, investigated the effects of CLA supplementation for 12 months. In the June 2004 *American Journal of Clinical Nutrition*, a study of 180 overweight (BMI 25-30) subjects reported that supplementation with CLA for one year resulted in lower body fat mass, greater lean body mass and, increased LDL (e.g. good cholesterol).[143] This is not the only study to report positive results. Science supports the theory that one or more of the naturally occurring CLA isomers can reduce body fat while enhancing lean body mass.[144]

How does CLA work? It may increase energy expenditure in its metabolism.[145] Or, CLA may suppress leptin levels.[146,147] The exact mechanism has not yet been determined. Of note, CLA is also claimed by researchers to have properties of being anti-cancer, anti-inflammatory and anti-atherogenic.[148]

The safety profile of CLA appears to be good. Animal trials suggest that CLA is safe,[149,150] at least in animals. Human trials have generally reported no significant side effects. However, it has been suggested that CLA may increase oxidative stress and insulin resistance.[151,152]

Where do you get this fat? CLA is a fat found in dairy milk and beef, and can be found in safflower and sunflower oil blend supplements.
Therefore, it appears that there are many fears and phobias about fat that are unfounded. It is not fat that makes us fat. In fact, some fat is good for us in preventing and treating some illnesses and

diseases. Next time you're at a friend's house party, be sure to mention that not all fat is bad, and that some fats can help you fight disease. Mention that fish is a great source of DHA and that can help you be smarter. Now that you know about fats, you'll be the smart one at the party.

Now, that we're all fat savvy and know that fat is not to blame for our problem with obesity, it is time to look further. On our quest to find a healthy diet we're now ready to take what we've learned and determine what a good diet is.

Chapter 6:
A "Good" Diet

What happened to us? Why are we so confused about what to eat? Firstly, we can blame it on our confusion about fat. Concerns in the early 1960s that North Americans were eating too much animal fat and cholesterol prompted doctors to begin recommending that patients reduce the amount of fat in their diets. However, as these recommendations failed to distinguish between the good and bad fats it ultimately created a phobia towards all fats. Yet, we all now know that good fats are fish and vegetable oils, known as unsaturated fats. Bad fats, such as trans and saturated fats, are associated with clogged arteries, heart disease, and other health problems. This misinformed fat phobia led to the first major food confusion of our generation in North American, and the first misdirection in our eating habits. We all believed that all fat is bad. Today, some still do.

Secondly, the introduction of anti-carbohydrate diets has made people question almost every food group of our diets. The carb craze has us questioning (i) the value of protein, (ii) the truth of the fat phobia and, (iii) the goodness of carbohydrates.

i) The carb craze questioning of protein has fueled the debate of whether the human body was designed to eat meat as a source of protein? Scientifically, the jury is still out on this issue. In the scientific community, some believe that humans

113

are well suited for a diet that is relatively high in protein and low in carbohydrates and, that such a diet is crucial to healthy insulin behavior.[153] Others are less sure of this argument,[154] believing that perhaps humans were not meant to be carnivores. To date, no conclusions can be made to whether we are supposed to eat meat or not.

ii) The fat phobia of our generation has also been questioned as low-carb diets have advertised that it's healthy to eat a diet high in protein, even suggesting that animal meat and other sources of saturated fat, previously thought to be very unhealthy foods, are part of this seemingly healthy diet. The coinciding research boom on essential fatty acids directly attacks the fat phobias by suggesting that there are fats that are essential to health. This and other factors have left many North Americans truly confused about fat, and where and how it should fit into a healthy diet.

iii) Obviously, the low-carb and anti-carb trend has resulted in consumer confusion about carbohydrates. Are they good? Are they bad? Many brands have hit the market recently advertising their low carbohydrate count, suggesting to consumers that this is a nutrient to be wary off. In fact, to date over 1500 new low-carb foods have appeared on supermarket shelves.[155] Also, it has been estimated that low-carb product sales will reach $30 billion in the U.S. in 2004, which is more than Coca-Cola sales worldwide. The result is a discrimination against total carbohydrates, as opposed to the glycemic index, or type of carbohydrate. Good carbs (complex) have low glycemic indexes and are foods with whole grains and/or are high in fibre. These foods are valuable to us and should not be discriminated against. It is that white, high glycemic index, highly processed carbohydrate we need to be wary of.

No matter who you are, these recent media attention has caused us to waver and question our belief in the recommendations given to us by our parents: three square meals a day, including meat, potatoes and a vegetable. Today we find ourselves wondering should the meat be beef or fish? Potato or whole wheat bread or none at all? We're confused. So, let's debunk the myths. We've looked at the science behind protein, carbohydrates and fat. We know what the facts are. Now, let's find a way to put the facts into an easy to understand, easy to follow dietary plan that can lead us to better and healthier living – a good, almost perfect diet.

a) A Good Low-Carb Diet

Some of you may still be wavering, unsure whether to take the plunge into the low-carbohydrate lifestyle. Therefore, in our attempt to find a good, almost perfect diet we need to determine if there is a good low-carb diet.

Through all of our investigating we seem to have discovered that there are some serious problems with the conventional low-carbohydrate diet; primarily the confusion between good and bad carbohydrates and secondly, the lack of vital nutrients that is associated with low-carbohydrate diets.

There are both good and bad carbohydrates. If a typical North American diet was our starting point, to get to a good low-carb diet, we would first remove white, processed carbohydrates. Such foods include white bread, most cereals, crackers, cookies, pastries, sugar candy and pop. By doing such, we have reduced the total amount of carbohydrates, and total amount of calories consumed. How do we fill in this gap? Instead of filling the gap with fatty foods and meats, reach for more vegetables and fruit, whole grain carbohydrates, beans and nuts. By doing such a simple exchange we have managed to reduce the amount of bad carbohydrates in the diet and, increase the amount of protein, fruits and vegetables consumed. Also, we have actually exchanged high calorie-low nutritional value foods (i.e. processed foods tend to contain extra fat and calories and lack nutrients), for lower calorie, more nutritionally valuable foods – an important factor to creating any healthy diet.

Now, for the lack of nutrients that can occur in the high protein/low-carbohydrate diets, we need to consider supplements. Many essential vitamins and minerals are lost in low-carbohydrate diets as these diets tend to remove fortified carbohydrates such as bread and cereals. Also, the reduced amount of fruits and vegetables, particularly in the anti-carb diets, emphasize the need to supplement with a multi-vitamin and mineral. Essential fatty acids are also a concern. The current North American diet does not contain sufficient omega fatty acids, nor does the newer high protein/low-carbohydrate diets. The value of essential fatty acids has already been discussed. Everyone should consider an essential fatty acid supplementation. In fact, the American Heart Association recommends that adults consume 900mg of omega-3s each day. Reach for a high quality essential fatty acid supplement, ideally with a proper ratio of omega-3 to omega-6 (2:1) to ensure that your body is getting all the needed essential nutrients as an important part of any diet, including a good low-carbohydrate diet.

These guidelines to a healthy low-carb diet are not just theories. Researchers are continually studying the effects of various diet combinations. In 2005, researchers reported in the *Journal of*

Nutrition, that a protein-rich diet may have its place in healthy weight loss plans. The trial involved 50 overweight women who all consumed the same number of calories and exercised regularly. However, one group substituted protein foods for high carbohyrated foods. In both groups of dieters, the exercise helped spare lean muscle tissue and target fat loss. But, the protein-rich, high-exercise group, lost even more weight, and almost 100 per cent of the weight loss was fat. In the high-carbohydrate, high-exercise group, however, as much as 25 to 30 per cent of the weight lost was muscle. *(Journal of Nutrition, 2005; 135(8):1903-10)* Thus, perhaps a good low-carb diet can be beneficial in adding weight loss.

b) What is a good diet?

What is a good diet? That is a very good question. Are there set criteria for a good diet? Some would say that a good diet is one that causes weight loss. However, for a diet to be good is there a criterion for the amount or the rate at which the diet causes weight loss? Or, is a good diet one that offers the body all of the elements it needs to be healthy, both in the sense of being resistant to disease and at a healthy weight. By investigating past diets, having been deemed good or bad, perhaps we can discover what a good diet is.

There have been many fad diets in the past few decades. Each of which has come and gone, proving to be yet another 'get-thin-quick' scheme for its victims who find themselves quickly gaining the weight back. In the past decade there have been a number of diets that have claimed to be the diets of all diets. Some of my favorites include the Cabbage Soup Diet, the Drinking Man's diet and the Hollywood 24 hour diet for their amusing theories and amazing followings by the North American public. Yet, each has come, gone and been deemed a failure. In our quest to find out what a good diet is, perhaps we can learn a few lessons from bad diets.

There was an article published in December 2003, in *Wired Magazine* titled, "The Thin Science of Fad Diets", that compared the fad diets of the time. The report was created using information from leaders in the dietary planning field. The article ranked the most popular diets of the year based on their scientific founding and likely ability to work. The Atkins diet was ranked the lowest as it was said to violate all food and nutrition science. The South Beach also ranked low as its 3 phase plan was said to encourage accelerated weight loss in the first phase, not a biologically healthy process, and its unfounded suggestion in the first phase to eat almost no carbs. The Eat Right for Your Blood type was said to not be founded on any science, and therefore also ranked low. The highest score was the Healthy Eating Pyramid from Harvard that encourages plant oil, plant products and whole grains. Also at the top of the charts was the Mediterranean diet which focuses on fruits, vegetables, fibre and lean meats.[156] Based on the results of these dietary planning field experts, it would appear that a good diet is one that focuses on ensuring sufficient consumption of foods that offer high nutritional value and that uses the current nutritional scientific knowledge. Most importantly, it appears that diets that encourage a well balanced mix of food groups are superior. One can also conclude that the Healthy Eating Pyramid and the Mediterranean diet warrant further investigation as they appear to have elements of good diets.

One aspect of the latest fad diets that has always puzzled me is the lack of focus on fruits and vegetables. Most diets are based on protein or carbohydrate consumption. Despite vast efforts by national produce marketing agencies to increase awareness of fruits and vegetables as part of a healthy diet, there is yet to be a diet designed just for them. These foods are high in fibre. Fibre makes us feel full fast. Fruits and vegetables are low in calories, and high in nutritional value. They are packed full of disease fighting compounds called antioxidants. Not to mention they are a source of calcium, potassium, magnesium, zinc and many other important minerals. What about vitamins? We all know that vitamins are the keys to many vital biological processes. Fruits and vegetables are the best source of most vitamins. All in all, fruits and vegetables are foods of very high nutritional value and perhaps a diet high in fruits and vegetables is a perfect diet for health and weight loss. Yes, weight loss. In fact, one of the most popular weight loss programs in North America, Weight Watchers, highlights fruits and vegetables as a key part of their diet by giving these foods a low point value, thereby enticing participants to eat more produce.

i) The Mediterranean and Healthy Eating Pyramid

Not surprisingly, the Mediterranean diet and the Healthy Eating Pyramid, the two top scoring diets according to leaders in the dietary planning field, highly encourage fruit and vegetable consumption. The older of the two, the Mediterranean diet, has been deemed by many to be the healthiest diet, particularly for the heart, that we know of to date. The Mediterranean diet has long been an integral part of dietary patterns around the world. It advocates that pasta is a vehicle for fruits, vegetables, nuts, whole grains and wines, which have low glycemic indices, carry healthful antioxidant benefits and are a source of fibre and omega-3 fatty acids. It suggests that protein-dense foods containing saturated fat be eaten only a few times a month. These types of food include beef. Also, at the top of the Mediterranean pyramid are sweets. Fruits, vegetables, legumes and beans are highly encouraged with this diet. Perhaps the best part of the Mediterranean diet is that it is easy to see the differentiation of the fats. Olive oil is given a separate section on the pyramid letting people know that this type of fat is acceptable. It also divides the protein sources into its appropriate categories of legumes and beans, fish, poultry, eggs and other meat (e.g. pork, beef). Unfortunately, this diet does fall short in that it lacks the separation of carbohydrates into high and low glycemic indices, or simple and complex carbohydrates. However, each of the foods emphasized in this diet (e.g. fish, fruits and vegetables, nuts and plant oils) has proven to be heart healthy.[157]

MEDITERRANEAN DIET PYRAMID

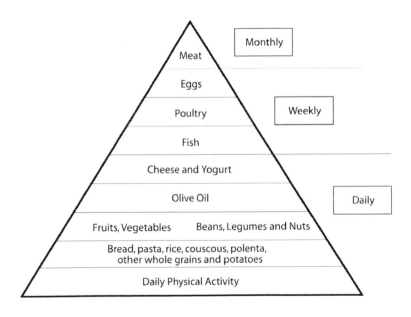

HEALTHY EATING PYRAMID

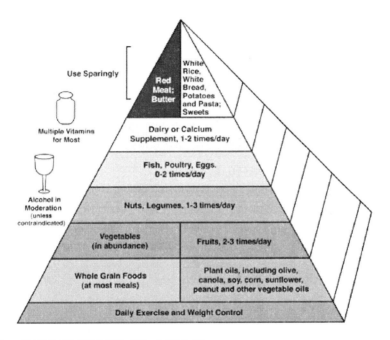

From EAT, DRINK, AND BE HEALTHY by Walter C. Willett, MD
copyright Simon & Schuster 2001.

As for the Healthy Eating Pyramid, this food guideline was created at Harvard in an attempt to correct what its scientists felt were problems with the United States Dietary Food Pyramid. The Healthy Eating Pyramid sits on a foundation of daily exercise and weight control. Next on the pyramid are whole grain foods, which are suggested to be eaten at most meals. This is because carbohydrates are the fuel of the body. They recommend that the best sources of carbohydrates are whole grains such as oatmeal, whole-wheat bread, and brown rice. This is great as they are focusing on low glycemic index, or complex carbohydrates.

121

At the next building block on the Healthy Eating Pyramid there are plant oils. As the average American gets one third or more of his or her daily calories from fats, it's not surprising that fats sit so close to the bottom of the pyramid. However, because they are plant fats or good fats, it encourages people to reach for foods that contain good fat and avoid those with bad fat. A possible fault of this pyramid is that fats come first and it takes so long to get to vegetables and fruits. However, at least the Healthy Eating Pyramid suggests that one eats vegetables in abundance and fruits two to three times a day. This encourages people to focus on vegetables, which tend to be eaten less in today typical diet, unlike the more portable and sweet fruits. Positively, this pyramid places more emphasis on nuts and legumes than fish, poultry and eggs. Then, surprisingly one finds dairy or calcium supplement close to the top of the pyramid despite the concerns of calcium deficiency diseases such as osteoporosis, and recent research that suggests that dairy may help to encourage weight loss in an energy restricted diet.[158]

At the top of the Healthy Eating Pyramid one finds red meat, butter, and the high glycemic index carbohydrates such as white rice, white bread, potatoes and sweets. This is good advice. Finally, beside the pyramid, giving it almost a feeling that it should be avoided, is a multi-vitamin. Contrary to this pyramid, a multi-vitamin has become a staple in dietary recommendations by dieticians across North America and perhaps is misrepresented in this pyramid.

Both the Mediterranean and the Healthy Eating Pyramid offer good advice about healthy eating. They both appear to put more emphasis on fruits and vegetables than other fad diets. They also separate proteins and fats into better and worse. However, the

Mediterranean fails to separate high and low glycemic indices and the Healthy Eating Pyramid places too much emphasis on fat and sends a potentially confusing message about supplements. However, we can see that we are getting closer to finding that good, almost perfect diet.

ii) The Portfolio Eating Plan

A more recent dietary eating program, designed by Dr. David Jenkins from the University of Toronto has caught some attention as being a good diet. It was designed initially to prove that a carefully constructed diet could lower cholesterol levels in humans as effectively as statins, a commonly prescribed pharmaceutical. In fact, in 2005, the *American Journal of Clinical Nutrition* published Dr. Jenkins' study which concludes that a diet rich in fibre, soy and vegetables lowers cholesterol just as much as statin drugs.[159] This plan is not as easily drawn out as the Healthy Eating Pyramid or the Mediterranean diet; however there are 4 key elements. First, snacks should include almonds. A daily handful or two is well supported in science as a heart healthy action. Second, viscous fibre should make up about 20g in a 2,000 calorie diet. Viscous fibre can be found in beans, such as kidney, lima, pinto and white, as well as in oats, strawberries, dried prunes, broccoli, chickpeas, barley, and grapefruit. Third, plant sterols from avocados, soybeans, olive and corn oil, chickpeas and almonds are important. Plant sterols are also available in natural supplements, such as beta-sitosterol. Fourth, is soy protein which is available as a powder, in milk drinks, as tofu and more thanks to recent developments in the food industry. One will notice that this diet does not include fast foods, white or high glycemic index carbohydrates, sweets or saturated fats. But, it does include a focus on high quality source of protein

123

such as beans and soy, and encourages a number of fruits and vegetables. The Portfolio Eating Plan is not necessarily the best diet as it is not very universal. However, it is a valuable diet for the thousands of North Americans who have elevated cholesterol levels and is therefore an important diet. In our quest for a good diet, we can learn from the Portfolio Eating Plan as it shows us that it is possible to use food as medicine and that one could truly eat a diet of all natural, unprocessed foods and be healthy. Also, this diet suggests perhaps a better terminology for a healthy diet – a plan. If society sees a diet as dietary regime that is restricted in calories, trend based, and causes quick weight loss, then perhaps diet is not the work we are looking for. Perhaps this book should have been entitled *The Search for a Good Plan.* It is important to recognize that the word diet can mean a calorie restricted, trendy weight loss regime as well as a plan of how to get healthy foods. Here we are searching for the diet plan.

iii) Raw Living

Living raw is the new old. It's the old way of eating that is becoming the latest new movement in healthy living. And, there are many reasons why it's worth looking at, as it encourages a lot of "good" diet principles.

We all know the disadvantages of eating processed foods: the lack of nutritional content, the addition of unnatural preservatives, trans fats, and sweeteners. There are enormous benefits to eating real, natural foods. Raw and living foods are foods that contain enzymes. Living foods contain more enzymes than raw foods. For example, a nut is a raw food as the nut is dormant. A sprouted nut is a living food as it is actively growing. The nut contains dormant enzymes. The sprouted nut contains only active enzymes. The idea of eating a raw and/or living diet is that you are eating foods in the state where they have the highest nutritional value.

The raw and living diet movement is gaining speed recently, but is based on very old theories. Looking back at the original diets of humans there was no drive-thrus, or bakeries. Our main food staple for centuries was fruits, vegetables, whole grains and nuts. To date, plant based foods are the most efficient and effective way for our bodies to get energy. This can be seen through the use of barley grass and other "green" foods as energy and immune boosters. Perhaps in another million years our bodies will have evolved enough to be able to properly identify and digest a French fry. For now a French fry is an unfamiliar item to our digestive systems and likely an ineffectively digested food item. We're best off eating raw or living foods when it comes to effective digestion.

What is a raw or living diet? A raw diet is one that contains foods in their raw state, or not cooked over a temperature of about 116 degrees Fahrenheit. At this temperature enzymes can become inactive. A raw or living foodist eats a diet of 75%+ living or raw (preferably organic) foods. Ideally, a raw diet is 100% raw and living foods. However, it is best for each person to determine what percentage is right for them.

What is the theory behind raw living? Firstly, raw and living foods are enzymatically active. Our digestive system has to create enzymes to break down the foods we eat. This is a very energy expending task. Enzymes that naturally occur in raw and living foods lower the amount of energy required for your body digest food. There are some who theorize that the extensive production of digestive enzymes needed to break down the highly processed North American diet may cause the pancreas to burn out leading to gastrointestinal illness. This is not supported to date by conclusive scientific research.

We're discussing the raw diet because it has some elements of a "good" diet. This includes a diet of raw foods naturally high in fibre. Fibre has many healthy benefits including helping reduce cholesterol levels, improving gastrointestinal health, bowel regularity and helps lower the glycemic load. Fibre also makes us feel full, reducing over eating. Also, this diet encourages eating lots of fruits and vegetables, well more than the recommended 10 a day. Of those many servings of vegetables and fruit, this raw diet encourages eating organically which is healthy as it lowers the potential amount of pesticides and herbicides consumed.

Raw foods are also very healthy as they are alkaline forming. Most of the foods we eat cause an acidic reaction in the blood. However, raw foods cause a basic of alkaline reaction. This is important as an acidic environment is thought to encourage disease such as osteoporosis. Scientists have been exploring the pH effect of food in various ways. There are a few general conclusions that can be made from the research to date. Firstly, the body has a pH of about 7.4. The body's functions cannot occur beyond pH values of 6.8 to 8. The higher the concentration of the ion, H+, the more acidic the pH. The ion, H+, is involved in many vital reactions and its balanced concentration is essential to life. Secondly, studies have shown that an acidic diet negatively affects calcium metabolism in the body resulting in skeletal calcium loss.[160] In other words, an acidic diet is not bone healthy.

126

Conclusively though the science on raw and living foods is lacking and therefore no conclusions can be made towards its potential to cause improvements in energy, digestion or reducing disease risks.

Before we move onto designing a good diet, let's take a quick look into calories. Calorie-counters is a name I give those of us who have spent part of our lives reading labels and adding up the total number of calories we consume in an attempt to keep a balance between intake and output. Now, please don't imagine a bunch of women running around all day with calculators in our pockets. We just know that weight management involves the balance between the total number of calories consumed minus the number of calories used in a day. The basic nutritional needs of most people are approximately 2,000 calories a day for women and 2,500 for men. However, people who are very active, such as manual laborers or professional athletes may need up to 4,000 calories a day or more. Pregnant women and nursing mothers require about 300-500 more calories/day than women who are neither pregnant nor nursing. An interesting fact, is that if you were to eat 100 calories more each day than you burn, (e.g. just 2 pieces of red licorice) you'd gain 10 pounds in a year. That may not seem like that much until you think about what might happen over 5 years; that's 50 pounds This does not mean that to be thin you have to count your calories at every turn. You simply have to be conscious that some foods have more calories than others and that you may want to take calories into consideration when you are picking which item to snack on. For example, if you have the choice between an apple and carrots with dip, as both have a good nutritional value you may want to waver towards the apple as it has fewer calories.

Most importantly, remember that the only scientifically proven and safe way to successfully lose weight is to have a daily caloric deficit of 500 calories.

c) A "Good" almost Perfect Diet

What is the perfect diet? Perhaps this question will plague us for centuries. To be honest, there is no perfect diet. There is no perfect diet for everyone. It would be presumptuous to assume that after our investigation of the pros and cons of the latest fad diets, and the current scientific knowledge, that we could create a perfect diet for everyone. Each person is unique in their dietary needs. We each have our own metabolic rate, allergies, food preferences and medical conditions. Therefore, it is important to realize that when discussing a "good" diet, it's a generalization of what a typical North American should be eating based on current scientific knowledge. Luckily, there are some key elements to a healthy diet that we can all use to create our own "good" and perhaps almost perfect diet.

Every diet is based on a different set of rules. However, as we've seen in our investigation of various food categories, and popular diets of our time, there are some key universal elements to healthy eating. Some of these universal elements can be seen in government dietary guidelines. In particular, the dietary guidelines of both the United States and Canada highly recommend a well balanced diet. This has been echoed throughout the research we've investigated.

What is a well balanced diet? What should we eat? Based on scientific data, there are many answers. Some of which are quite complicated, involving the combination of various types of foods, the elimination of some foods, the time of day to eat, and more. Therefore, let's discuss some simple ways to work on changing your diet into a healthier one. By taking small steps, we can work our way into a healthier diet in an almost effortless way.

Why should one make dietary changes slowly? Our dietary choices and patterns have been formed through our daily activities, timelines and habits. Also, the food choices of our parents, children and partners have influenced the groceries we buy, the meals we serve and the way we cook. These are all habits that have taken a long time to form, and therefore will be hard to break if we want to change them for the long-term. Therefore, by changing our diets slowly, we're more likely to make the change successfully and sustain it.

It's time to unveil the most important rule of healthy eating. This rule will be the first deciding factor as to whether a food item should or should not be eaten. The rule to a healthy diet: "Eat high nutrition value food." It's that easy. Now, what is a nutritionally valuable food? First, look at a food you're about to eat. Is it full of bad fat, (saturated or trans fat) and simple sugar? Has it been processed? If the answer is "no" to both of these questions than this food item is likely of high nutritional value. Next, ask is this food item a source of protein, good(complex) carbohydrates, vitamins and/or minerals? Hopefully, the answer is yes, as this means that this food is of high nutritional value. Pick foods that have a lot of nutrition packed into them. Unprocessed, whole foods have more nutrients naturally, than processed foods.

To better understand this concept of high nutritional value foods, let's try a few examples. You have the choice between a bean salad and an iceberg salad. Are they full of bad fat, simple sugar or processed? No. Is it a good source of protein, carbohydrates, vitamins and minerals? Yes, the vegetables are a source of good carbohydrates, minerals and vitamins. However, the bean salad is also a source of protein, and contains more fibre, vitamins and minerals than the iceberg lettuce salad. So, the more nutritionally valuable choice is the bean salad.

Let's try another example. You are to choose between a piece of wild salmon, and chicken cordon bleu. Are they full of bad fat and simple sugar? The salmon is not, but the chicken does have added saturated fat in the cheese middle. Are they a source of protein, good carbohydrates, vitamins and/or minerals? Both are sources of protein. However, since the chicken has added cheese, it is higher in bad fat. Yet, cheese is a source of calcium. This example is harder, as to determine if the cheese is a pro or a con, we have to look at the bigger picture. What else did you eat today, and what else are you eating with this meal? Are there better sources of calcium in your diet, such as green leafy vegetables and low-fat dairy products? If yes, than the salmon may be a better choice for this meal. If no, than perhaps you need the added calcium of the chicken. On the other hand, have you had omega-3s in your diet lately? If no, than the salmon is your best choice. It's important to realize that your diet is not just the meal you are about to eat, but the whole of what you've consumed over a few days. Balance out your key needs: protein, carbohydrates, good fats, calcium, vitamins, minerals, antioxidants. A balanced diet is a "good", healthy diet.

Excellent. Now, that we understand what high nutritional value foods are, we can move onto our easy steps towards a "good" diet. Firstly, and most importantly, we need to understand that change does not happen over night. No, it takes years to change your dietary patterns as these patterns took years to develop. It may mean venturing down a different aisle at the grocery store, or seeking out a good health food store in your city. Regardless, try these 16 tips to lead to healthier eating. Start with the first tip. When you tackle it, add the next. Some are designed that once you tackle the first, the second helps you move on. For example, if you tackle snacking correctly, you're already working on the next step of eating 5 to 10 servings of fruits and vegetables a day. Try not to skip any steps or rush through this process. This is not a diet – this is a plan to develop healthy eating, a "good" diet, and perhaps an almost perfect diet.

1) Eat breakfast.

In fact, make sure you eat at least 3 meals a day. You need fuel to function - particularly in the morning. In the morning, your body has been sleeping for 6 to 8 hours. It's low on sugar or glucose. It needs a kick start. It's an empty tank of gas. In the morning, you may have not eaten for up to 12 hours. Try that in the middle of the day and you'll be craving food. You may not feel hungry but your body will work much better if you eat breakfast. Also, people who eat breakfast are significantly less likely to be obese and diabetic than those who usually do not. The obesity and insulin resistance syndrome rates were 35% and 50% lower among people who eat breakfast every day compared to those who frequently skipped it.[161] So, get up and eat in the morning. What to eat for breakfast? Definitely eat some fruit or fruit juice, some complex carbohydrates and preferably a good source of protein, such as a soy cereal or a homemade breakfast shake with soy protein. Need a good morning shake recipe? See the Sample Diet and Recipes for my favorite morning fuel-up drink.

2) Avoid processed foods.

Despite their convenience they are always full of fat. That is why they taste so good. In particular, they tend to contain trans fats which are the evil of all bad fats. Cut out frozen dinners, crackers, cookies, chips and minute-ready side dishes. Even hot chocolate mix and children's cereals are full of trans fats and other unhealthy ingredients. Packaged and processed foods can be full of fat, sodium and other ingredients your body does not need. Challenge yourself to read the side panel of packaged foods in your cupboard. Watch for trans fat, saturated fat, cholesterol, sodium, hydrogenated vegetable oil, shortening or artificial sweeteners like aspartame as ingredients. None of these ingredients are valuable to a healthy diet and should be avoided. And, be wary of packaged vegetables – be sure they don't have added preservative chemicals. The best foods are not in packages – plus, using less packaging is earth friendly.

3) Snack right.

Stop eating a chocolate bar because you're hungry at 4 o'clock, or running to the donut store at 10 o'clock for that mid-morning fix. These foods are full of simple sugar and bad fat. The donuts and chocolate bars of the world give you a big rush of glucose that makes you irritable, and then the rush disappears rapidly leaving you flat and feeling awful. In fact, some people say that the sugar and bad fat roller-coaster leaves them craving the next high simple sugar, bad fat food to get them feeling high again. It becomes like a drug. Instead, reach for nuts, fruit, or a handful of vegetables when you have those hunger rumblings at 10 and 4. Also, try low fat yogurt, nut or peanut butter, or a hummus spread. These high protein-low fat foods are more nutritionally valuable and will make you feel full and with no hidden tricks.

Allison's Favorite Stomach Rumbling Snacks
   a.   a handful of almonds
   b.   trail mix
   c.   an apple, pear, plum, orange, all fruits
   d.   hummus and whole wheat pita
   e.   low fat yogurt with granola and berries
   f.   dried fruit bars (organic)
   g.   a small bowl of high-protein cereal with fruit
   h.   baby carrots, plum tomatoes, raw broccoli and cauliflower

4)   Eat 5 to 10 servings of fruits and vegetables per day.
Fruits and vegetables are great snacks. They fit well in lunches and come in so many colours and sizes. It's important to eat a variety of vegetables and fruits as each colour represent a different set of antioxidants, or damage fighters that your body needs to stave off disease and illness. When you eat 10 servings of a variety of fruits and vegetables you'll notice that you get sick less, and you feel full sooner, with less desire to snack on unhealthy foods. Also, this satiety resulting from fruit and vegetable consumption can result in weight loss for some, as vegetables and fruit are low in calories. Fruits and vegetables are well known for their ability to reduce the risk of cancer and heart disease. In Canada, there is an approved health claim stating just that; "A diet rich in a variety of vegetables and fruit may reduce the risk of some types of cancer." In the United States there is an approved health claim noting the ability of a diet high in vegetables and fruits to reduce the risk of heart disease. "Diets low in

saturated fat and cholesterol and rich in fruits, vegetables, and grain products that contain some types of dietary fiber, particularly soluble fiber, may reduce the risk of heart disease, a disease associated with many factors."

The fibre content of fruits and vegetables are also a great reason to eat them as they can help with regularity. Challenge yourself to eat 10 servings everyday for a week. It's easier than you think. Just pack an apple, some baby carrots and/or plum tomatoes, raisins, celery sticks, a cut grapefruit, a berry mix or even natural, unsweetened apple sauce to your lunch. If you snack on fruits and vegetables, and eat at least one serving each meal, you'll quickly find your eating 5-8 servings already. Just up the size of your salads, add another vegetable to dinner or drink a glass of juice at breakfast and you'll easily reach that goal of 10 servings a day.

5) Exercise

Now that your diet is starting to take shape we need to kick it up a notch – literally. A healthy lifestyle includes daily exercise. Your muscles want to shake and move. They love to be worked – so give those legs a kick. Simple things like taking a 15 minute walk at a break at work can help. Have your family start 30 minute evening walks. Take the kids tobogganing, or for a bike ride. Join a yoga, dance or tai chi class. Get involved in a league have it be baseball, volleyball or ultimate Frisbee. Or, join the local gym and take a friend to get you there, or go to the classes and meet some new people. What ever it is, be active. Exercise is a very important part of a healthy diet plan. Make sure each day you do something active. Once you've tackled this, try to pump up 3 of your exercises to include either weights, or cardiovascular exercise. Get your heart rate up or make those muscles burn and you'll see big changes in your body and there'll be a huge increase in your energy levels. Be active and you'll get a healthy addiction to healthy active living.

6) Eat your vegetables first, then your protein and last your carbohydrates.

When sitting at the dinner table give your body what it needs most first – vegetables and protein. Then, if you are still hungry, eat the carbohydrates on your plate. You'll notice that instead of leaving salad on your plate, you'll leave potatoes, bread or rice; items that are of lower nutritional value than the vegetables you used to leave. This veggies-first concept is not just a silly rule from my kitchen to yours. A study in the *Journal of the American Dietetic Association* compared what happens when you eat a meal with a salad and a meal without. They found that eating a large salad (3 cups) before a meal lowered the overall caloric intake of the meal by up to 12%, compared to eating no salad.

7) Eat slower.

According to the *European Journal of Clinical Nutrition*, it takes about 20 minutes after you start eating to feel full.[162] If you eat more slowly you will reach 20 minutes before you've scoffed down the extra side of French fries and large piece of chocolate cheese cake that you really didn't need. This also supports our eat vegetables and protein first concept. If you eat vegetables and protein first, you'll be close to your 20 minutes once you hit the carbohydrates, and you'll naturally reduce your carbohydrate consumption. This is a healthier way to lower your carbohydrate consumption than the no-carb or anti-carb philosophy discussed earlier.

135

8) If you tend to eat a lot of carbohydrates, focus on adding in new high nutritional value protein sources to your diet.

How about nuts as your mid-afternoon snack, instead of crackers or a bag of potato chips? How about yogurt for a snack? Find recipes that contain beans in them and add these to your dinners. Take a bean salad for lunch, or tuna and toast or no-trans fat crackers. Good sources of protein such as fish, soy, nuts and beans will fill you up faster, give you lots of energy and are low in fat. Focus on these fab-four protein sources and you'll be better off. If you still like the idea of snack bars, visit your local health food store and look for a raw food bar that contains no trans fat and is high in fibre and protein. These bars will be organic and full of natural ingredients, meaning their likely to be the healthiest protein bar on the shelf.

9) Pick appropriate proportions.

Big portions encourage people to eat more. Furthermore, eating big portions of calorie dense foods (e.g. biggie sized fries) boosts calorie consumption even farther. Unfortunately, this type of big calorie eating does not provide any additional satisfaction according to research. Research has found that calorie density and portion size add together to affect caloric intake.[163] In other words, eating large portions of calorie-rich foods has been found to increase the total number of calories consumed which is not healthy and can lead to obesity. Yet, we still eat calorie-rich food because it seems to calm the nerves. However, eating too much can lead to obesity, depression and stress.[164] American adults, who are notorious for being big portion lovers, have recently reported that restaurants have gone too far. In a recent survey, 53% of American adults reported that portions are

136

too large at restaurants.[165] So, be portion wary. If it is a high calorie food, eat less.

10) Get your Essential Fatty Acids.
North Americans are deficient in their omega fatty acids. Try to eat 2 servings of fish a week. A serving is about the size of a deck of cards or the palm of your hand. Your best sources of omega-3 fatty acids are salmon, tuna, mackerel, sardines and anchovies. Taking a good quality omega-3 fatty acid supplement is another option. Or, better yet use a omega 3,6,9 combination that uses organic flax, fish and borage oil as these will give you an optimal dose of omega 3 (ALA, EPA and DHA) and omega 6 (LA and GLA). Ensuring your body has the needed essential fatty acids (e.g. LA and ALA) to function properly may help reduce your risk of North America's top diseases including heart disease, cancer, arthritis, depression, Alzheimer's and menopause. See the previous chapter on fats for all the details on essential fatty acids.
If you're major interest is to lose weight, then look into the fatty acid called conjugated linoleic acid (CLA). CLA appears to help maintain a healthy body weight, as it may help reduce body fat and increase lean muscle mass. Health benefits attributed to CLA include reducing the risk of cancer, heart disease, arthritis and the onset of diabetes.[166]

11) Take a multivitamin.
Across North America doctors and dieticians recommend taking a multivitamin to ensure adequate intake of all needed vitamins and minerals. No matter how much of a rainbow you try to get onto your plate, we can all miss a vitamin or two. A good quality multivitamin will contain a

variety of all the essential vitamins to help ensure that your body has all the right elements it needs to function right. Did you know that vitamins are key factors in many of the body's reactions? For example, vitamin B6, B12 and folate are key elements required in the body to keep homocysteine levels low. High homocysteine is a risk factor for arthrosclerosis, a form of heart disease. Therefore, all vitamins and minerals are important to your body's health, so be sure you're getting an adequate intake.

12) Eat Greens.

Foods that are green are really important as they offer a complete range of vitamins, minerals, fibre, antioxidants and amino acids to help your body run smoothly. Some animals only eat greens foods, such as rabbits. They're quick, cute and can see well. Not bad traits for us to have too.

Also, green foods such as barley grass, contain active enzymes like superoxide dismutase (SOD). This enzyme is an antioxidant, meaning that it prevents oxidation in the body that leads to damage and disease. SOD has been implicated in many important biological reactions and has been suggested as an important anti-aging enzyme. So, eat those greens. Have broccoli, kale, spinach, bok choy, brussel sprouts, green peas, barley grass, wheat grass and sprouts and stock up on SOD for healthy living.

13) Calcium.

Most sources of calcium are also sources of saturated fat and cholesterol. Thus, you can find yourself lacking calcium if you're trying to avoid food sources with bad fat. Calcium is involved in and needed for every muscle contraction in your body. Every time you breathe, the muscles involved only work because calcium is present. Therefore, it is very important that your diet contains sufficient calcium. If your diet is low in calcium, the body will pull calcium from your bones to compensate. If this occurs over a long term you're increasing the risk of osteoporosis. So, be sure to get lots of calcium for overall health and strong bones.

Also, The Quebec Family Study of 235 men and 235 women concluded that there is a correlation between levels of dietary calcium and body composition.[167] This is in accordance with other research that increasing calcium intake may decrease fat formation and reduce body weight and obesity. So be sure to have adequate calcium intake in your diet to help attain that healthy waist line.

Calcium supplements come in many forms. The most recent media wave suggested that coral calcium is the most absorbable form of calcium available. Coral calcium contains a naturally high percentage of calcium to magnesium (i.e. about 2 to 1). This is why it is thought to be a beneficial supplement, as this high ratio likely maximizes the amount absorbed in the body. This was based on a single study.[168] Of the more historical calcium supplements, calcium carbonate is the most well known because it is more concentrated and, therefore, requires that a smaller number of pills be taken. However, calcium citrate is thought to have a more appealing pH for absorption in the body and, has been shown in a recent study to be better at reducing bone re-absorption than calcium carbonate.[169] A lesser known calcium supplement, hydroxyapatite, is a form of calcium found naturally in bone tissue. It is therefore not suitable for vegans. Little research has been done to compare hydroxyapatite to calcium carbonate or citrate; however, it is thought to be an absorbable source as it contains naturally occurring minerals and vitamins, such as vitamin C, D and K. All in all, the scientific jury is still out on which calcium supplement is superior. However it does appear that sufficient magnesium and vitamin D are required for optimal calcium absorption.

14) Antioxidants

Imagine the ability to prevent aging and damaging events that can lead to disease. You can with antioxidants. These little warriors scavenge the body looking for free radicals, naturally occurring elements that are reactive and can cause damage that we associate with disease and aging. There are many types of antioxidants available today. Each is popular because it offers a different antioxidant, or has been shown in research to be helpful for a particular disease. For example, the plant wax policosanol is well known as a heart health antioxidant. Alpha lipoic acid is popular as it is the universal antioxidant because it can dissolve into both fat and water allowing it to penetrate the whole body. Also, alpha lipoic acid is capable of regenerating several other antioxidants back to their active states, including vitamin C, vitamin E, glutathione and coenzyme Q10. Grape seed extract contains a class of compounds called proanthocyanidins, which are potent free radical scavengers and appears to work with vitamin C to help the immune system. Lutein is from the carotenoid family and thought to be an important antioxidant for eye health. Lycopene is from tomatoes and has been shown in studies to be helpful for the prostate. There are many more antioxidants, each with its own special function. Choose the one or ones that suit your individual needs.

15) Consider chromium.

People who are concerned about carbohydrates because of their need to control their insulin levels should consider chromium. Chromium is an essential mineral thought to enhance insulin sensitivity. According to the Continuing Survey of Food Intakes by Individuals (1994-1996),[170] American diets are inadequate in the essential mineral chromium. Low intake may be associated with insulin resistance. Wheat, cooked peas, cheese, liver, egg and margarine are dietary sources of chromium.

16) Be Good to Your Gut

Healthy living is all about feeling healthy. With these dietary changes you may be noticing a change in your gastrointestinal tract. The increase in fibre will have you feeling more regular and less bloated. Now, consider taking the next step and look into probiotics. Probiotics are the good bacteria (e.g. flora) in your gut. Probiotics help improve the health of the intestinal tract by interacting with the cells of the gut lining and encouraging healthy behaviour including mucus production and proper immune function. Some of these healthy functions can inhibit the ability of bad bacteria from attacking and living in the gut.[171] This is perhaps the most promising part of probiotics.

Firstly, one needs to understand that there are different strains of probiotics. Most commonly known is the *Lactobicillus* and *Bifidus* bacterium family of species. In these families there are a number of species such as *Lactobicillus acidophilus* and *Lactobicillus casei*. There are some strains that have been shown in scientific studies to inhibit Candida growth (i.e. bad flora that causes yeast infections). Others are thought to inhibit E.Coli and other diarrhea causing bacteria from colonizing in the gut. There has been great success with probiotics use in children with diarrhea. On-going research is looking into the ability of probiotics to positively affect the immune system and therefore help with many diseases including vaginitis, lung diseases, cancer and more. Stay tuned for more on these good bacteria.

Probiotics can be helped by prebiotics. Prebiotics are food sources that probiotics use to grow and colonize. An example of a prebiotic is fructoogliosaccharide, or FOS. FOS is found in many foods and as a supplement.

Probiotic supplements are available in yogurts or dairy drinks at lower doses, or at high dosages in capsule form as a single strain, multiple strain or multiple species combination. To date, all forms appear to offer beneficial effects. However, a review study has suggested that it is possible that the multiple strain supplements offer the best effect.[172] To date, it is not conclusive as to which strain is best for which condition. However, it is certain that for a beneficial biological effect to occur the dosage of probiotic should be 10^9 cfu, or one billion bacteria.

From what we have seen, a "good" diet is one that is full of high nutritionally valuable food. Cut out low value foods such as processed foods, junk food and foods latent with bad fat (saturated and trans). Focus on natural, whole foods as they tend to be full of nutritional value. Most importantly, a good diet is one that is balanced. Be sure to eat all food groups in moderation and consult a qualified medical professional for personalized help in creating a good diet for you.

These 15 steps to a "good" diet will help you cut out unnecessary, low nutritional value foods, seek out more high nutritionally valuable foods, and ensure that you are getting the needed nutrients through food and supplements. These 15 steps are not going to ensure weight loss. However, many people find that once they move to a healthier diet that includes exercise, they naturally have a slow and gradual weight loss (the healthy kind of weight loss) until they reach their body's preferred weight. By eating a diet high in nutritional value, you feel full sooner and longer, eat less unnecessary calories and have a stronger immune system and healthier body.

CONCLUSIONS

The World Health Organization lists obesity among the top 10 health concerns in the world. In other words, obesity sits among AIDs as a great global health concern. The need for effective weight loss is not just great, but colossal. Our need to find a healthy diet that promotes a healthy weight is immense. Such need for diets explains the success of the numerous fad diets North America has seen over the past three decades. Among these fad diets, is the most recent, low-carbohydrate diets the answer? Is the high-protein, low-carbohydrate diet the be-all, end-all of diets? Perhaps a better question: Is a high protein/low-carb diet an effective way to attain weight loss? Evidence appears to vary. Some say yes, while others say no. It does appear to be effective for quick weight loss; however, it is uncertain as to whether high-protein/low-carb diets are either safe or useful for long term weight loss.

Therefore, should one do a high-protein/low-carbohydrate diet? A meta-analysis (i.e. review by scientists of all the research) on low-carbohydrate diets concluded that there is insufficient evidence to make recommendations for or, against the use of low-carbohydrate diets. A conclusion we can make after our review of these diets and, the science behind them is that there really are good carbohydrates, and bad carbohydrates. Differentiating between these types of carbohydrates appears to be important in having a healthy diet.

As asked at the beginning of this manuscript, what is the truth about carbs? The truth is that we need carbohydrates. They are our fuel. Some carbohydrates are better than others and there needs to be differentiation between them. Good carbohydrates, such as those that are whole grains and high in fibre are best and are supported by both science and long term diets, such as the Mediterranean diet as being a healthy choice. We should avoid white breads, white sugar and juices as these can cause high glucose peaks in the blood stream. Focus on high nutritional quality foods in your diet and you'll enjoy better health.

We have also discovered through our investigation of various diets of our time, that a well-balanced diet that is higher in good quality protein than the typical North American diet, and reduced in the intake of simple carbohydrates is supported by the science to date as being a good diet. In fact, we've discovered that a diet full of produce, whole wheat carbohydrates, low-fat protein sources, and a healthy schedule of exercise is the perfect start to a "good", almost perfect diet. Most importantly, we've learned that each person is different and we need to use variations of these "good" diet rules to attain a healthy weight.

Are we done with high protein/low-carbohydrate diets? In my opinion, we're likely not. When will we be done with diets all together? That is a question only time will tell. Hopefully, we can learn as a society to accept that we are all different. Each of us is made up of a different combination of genes. These genes determine who we are, what we look like and, to a degree, what weight we will be. We are not all meant to be runway models. However, we can learn to lead lifestyles that are healthier for us, thereby helping us attain healthy body weights. Exercise, stress reduction and, a healthy diet are important to vitality.

Maybe we are almost there. Perhaps, we are starting to recognize that it is not another diet that we need, but a change in our philosophy of what a healthy lifestyle is. For example, McDonald's, the largest fast food chain in the world, has chosen to make some healthier options on their menu. As a result they reported a 13.9% increase in sales. Also, cracker companies in North America have changed their manufacturing process to reduce and, in some cases, eliminate the presence of trans fatty acids in their foods. Also, in the wake of the trans fat movement of 2004, the Partnership for Essential Nutrition was founded to help educate Americans about the need for healthy carbohydrates. These actions and others offer a glimmer of hope that we, as a society, are ready to make changes to a healthier philosophy on food. No more quick fixes. Bring on the healthier foods. Perhaps, we are ready for healthier eating. However, it will take much more than a change in the value meal menu at the local fast food restaurant, and a change of fat content in crackers to fix our current societal dietary problems.

Yet, there is hope. There is hope that we are taking steps in the right direction. With each new piece of science discovered and, with each new bit of knowledge we become smarter and healthier. Because, with knowledge comes the power to live healthier lives.

Appendix

Protein Metabolism Charts:

Example at:

http://www.elmhurst.edu/~chm/vchembook/5900verviewmet.html

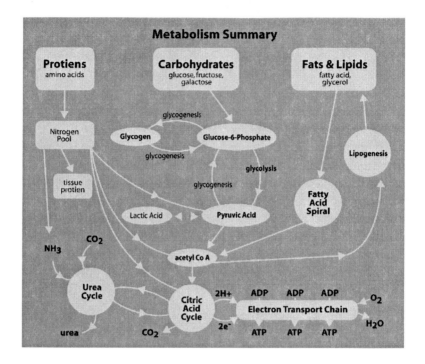

Glycemic Index:

GLYCEMIC INDEXES OF COMMON FOODS

Foods listed from highest to lowest glycemic index within category. Glycemic index was calculated using glucose as the reference with GI of 100. Modified from Foster-Powell and Brand Miller (1995).

Breads & Grains
waffle - 76
doughnut - 76
bagel - 72
wheat bread, white - 70
bread, whole wheat - 69
cornmeal - 68
bran muffin - 60
rice, white - 56
rice, instant - 91
rice, brown - 55
bulgur - 48
spaghetti, white - 41
whole wheat - 37
wheat kernels - 41
barley - 25

Cereals
Rice Krispies - 82
Grape Nuts Flakes - 80
corn Flakes - 77
Cheerios - 74
shredded wheat - 69
Grape Nuts 67
Life - 66
oatmeal - 61
All Bran - 42 **Fruits**
watermelon - 72
pineapple - 66
raisins - 64

banana - 53
grapes - 52
orange - 43
pear - 36
apple - 36

Starchy Vegetables
potatoes, baked - 83
potatoes, instant - 83
potatoes, mashed - 73
carrots - 71
sweet potatoes - 54
green peas - 48

Legumes
baked beans - 48
chick peas - 33
butter beans - 31
lentils - 29
kidney beans - 27
soy beans - 18

Dairy
ice cream - 61
yogurt, sweetened - 33
milk, full fat - 27
milk, skim - 32 **Snacks**
rice cakes - 82
jelly beans - 80
graham crackers - 74

corn chips - 73
life savers - 70
angel food cake - 67
wheat crackers - 67
popcorn - 55
oatmeal cookies - 55
potato chips - 54
chocolate - 49
banana cake - 47
peanuts - 14

Sugars
honey - 73
sucrose - 65
lactose - 46
fructose - 23

Beverages
soft drinks - 68
orange juice - 57
apple juice - 41

Sample Diet and Recipes:

To help in your transition to healthier eating below you will read about three practical examples of how one can use the tips given in the section on a Good Diet. This is not a perfect diet for all; however some may find these practical suggestions helpful in planning out how to achieve a diet high in fruits and vegetables, complex carbohydrates and good sources of protein.

Day 1:

o *Breakfast*
- 1 cup of Oatmeal with 1/4 cup of fresh blueberries
- 1 cup of juice (preferable organic)
- Handful of supplements (calcium, multivitamin, essential fatty acids (369), antioxidants, probiotic).

o *Mid-morning Snack*
- bowl of fresh fruit, or an apple, pear, plum, etc
- 1 L of bottled water

o *Lunch*
- organic bean minestrone soup
- carrot sticks and plum tomatoes
- no fat yogurt or probiotic yogurt

o *Mid-afternoon Snack*
- handful of almonds
- a piece of fruit
- 1L of water

o *Dinner*
- baked salmon with lemon and dill or rosemary topping
- wild rice
- slightly steamed broccoli
- bruschetta on whole grain bread lightly toasted with olive oil

Day 2

o *Breakfast*
- *Morning Start-Up Shake (see recipe at end of section)*
- Handful of supplements (calcium, multivitamin, essential fatty acids (369), antioxidants, probiotic).

o *Mid-morning Snack*
- homemade bran and blueberry muffin
- 1L of bottled water

o *Lunch*
- hummus dip and whole wheat bread or pita
- green leafy salad with a rainbow of vegetables

o *Mid-afternoon Snack*
- dried organic fruit bar
- 1L of water

o *Dinner*
- whole wheat crust pizza with pesto, roasted red pepper, red onion, spinach and pine nuts

- mixed bean salad
- fruit for dessert if needed

Day 3

o *Breakfast*
- Flax pancakes topped with fresh fruit
- Handful of supplements (calcium, multivitamin, essential fatty acids (369), antioxidants, probiotic).
- glass of organic fruit juice

o *Mid-morning Snack*
- dry roasted soya nuts

o *Lunch*
- Green leafy salad with sesame and sunflower seeds, lots of colourful vegetables, and half baked chicken breast)

o *Mid-afternoon Snack*
- Organic raw sprout bar

o *Dinner*
- Sushi with lots of raw vegetables
- Misu soup
- spinach and seasame seed salad

Allison's Morning Start-Up Shake
> 1/2 cup fruit juice of choice
> 1/2 cup frozen fruit
> 1/2 cup skim milk
> 1 banana
> 2-3 tbsp soy protein

2 tbsp Essential 3-6-9 fatty acids

2 tsp Organic Barley Grass

2 tbsp milled flax seed

Directions: Add all ingredients into blender. Blend until smooth. Serves 2-3.

Bean Salad

1 can of rinsed mixed beans

1/4 - 1/2 cup of chopped red onion

1 cup of fresh green beans

1 cup of fresh yellow beans

1 cup of organic extra-virgin Olive oil

1/2 cup of balsamic vinegar

dash of herbs of choice (e.g. thyme, pepper and garlic)

Directions: Mix all beans together. Combine oil, vinegar and herbs together in separate bowl. Pour over beans.

Pesto Pizza

1 bunches of washed fresh basil leafs

1/2 cup of olive oil

1/4 cup of light parmesan cheese

1 clove of chopped garlic

Whole wheat pizza crust, or pita

1/2 cup sliced red peppers

1/2 cup diced red onions

1/2 cup washed baby spinach leaves

1/2 cup of cheese of choice (e.g. goat cheese)

Directions: Blend basil, oil, cheese and garlic in blender. Pour over whole wheat crust. Roast peppers for about 2 minutes on stove top. Add pepper to pizza. Add onions, spinach and cheese to pizza as desired. Broil at 400 degrees for 10-15 minutes until cheese is melted or pizza browns. If crust is not pre-cooked, cook pizza according to pizza instructions.

Orange Bran Flax Muffins

1-1/2 cup oat bran
1 cup flour (try whole wheat)
1 cup milled or ground flax seed
1 cup natural bran
1 tbsp baking powder
1/2 tsp salt
2 whole oranges (washed quartered and seeded)
1 cup brown sugar
1 cup buttermilk (or skim milk)
1/2 cup olive oil
2 eggs
1 tsp baking soda
1-1/2 cup raisins (or try chocolate, or nuts)

Directions: In a large bowl, combine oat bran, flour, flax seed, bran, baking powder and salt. Set aside. In a blender, mix oranges, brown sugar, buttermilk, oil, eggs and baking soda. Blend well. Pour orange mixture into dry ingredients. Mix until well blended. Stir in raisins. Fill paper lined muffin tins almost to the top. Bake at 375 degrees for about 18 to 20 minutes. Cool in tins for 5 minutes before removing to cooling rack.

Banana and Fruit Breakfast Cookies

3 riped bananas
1 cup chopped Purely Bulk apricots or prunes
1/3 cup organic olive oil

2 cups Purely Bulk organic rolled oats
1/2 cup of Purely Bulk sunflower seeds
1 tsp vanilla
1/4 cup Herbal Select Milled Flax Seed

Makes 24, 1-1/2 inch breakfast cookies. Mash the bananas and combine with the chopped fruit and oil. Add the remaining ingredients and mix well. Drop by spoonfuls onto a greased cookie sheet, and flatten with a fork. Bake at 375° F for about 10-15 minutes, or until slightly browned.

Creamy Garlic Salad Dressing
1/4 cup water
1 medium sized crushed garlic clove
4 ounces soft tofu
1/4 cup Essential Fatty acid (369) oil
3 tablespoons lemon juice
2 tsp rice vinegar
1 tsp kelp (optional)
1 tbsp poppy seed
1 tsp dried dill weed
sea salt to taste

Directions: Combine all ingredients in a blender or food processor and process until smooth. Add milled flax seed as a variation.

Apple Zucchini Flax Pancakes

1 cup whole wheat flour
1/3 cup milled flax seed
3 tbsp beet or turbinado sugar

1 tbsp baking powder
1/2 tsp sea salt
1/4 tsp cinnamon
1/2 tsp nutmeg
2 eggs, separated, whites stiffly beaten
1-1/4 cup milk
3 tbsp oil
1/2 cup shredded apple
1/2 cup shredded zucchini

Directions: In a large bowl combine dry ingredients. In a medium bowl lightly beat together egg yolks, milk and oil. Add liquid to dry and stir only until combined. Shred apple and zucchini add to batter until combined. Fold in eggs whites. Preheat pan to medium heat and lightly grease. Using 1/3 cup measure yields 12 pancakes.

Product Guide:

Need help once you get to the store shelves? There are so many types of products available on the market. How do you tell which ones to buy? Here you will find some easy elements to look for on a package that can quickly tell you some basic important features of the product. Next, you'll find some product brands that are known for their quality and have a good reputation. Also, there are websites included to help you learn more about healthy food products in your continual transition to improve your diet. These will hopefully get you started in your quest to find a good diet that includes natural foods and supplements.

a) Certifications
Food products can be certified by various third party organizations with respect to being organic, kosher and more. Look for small official symbols on the front of packages that indicate the product is verified by a third party for its claimed health features. For example, commonly an organic product will show it is certified by showing the USDA or other certifying body on its package.

a) Health Claims
A claim on the front of the package can help you quickly recognize what feature may be of interest to you in the product. For example, if a product is high in fibre it will have a fibre content of about five grams or more.

Of note, the United States and Canada do not always agree on health claims. Therefore, on either side of the border one will find varying allowed health claims. Be a little skeptical when reading

161

claims to ensure you are really eating what you want to be eating. Be a wise consumer and read the Nutritional Facts panel and Ingredient listing to be sure that the health claim on the front of the package is supported by the products' hard facts. If in doubt, call the manufacturer of the product and ask them. Being health claim savvy can help you determine the potential health benefits of the product.

c) Nutritional Facts Panel

Each product is made with different ingredients and thus each food product will have a unique amount of calories, fats and carbohydrates. Be sure to read the ingredient panels on foods before you buy them. Watch out for trans fat, saturated fat and cholesterol as these are bad fats, or those that should be limited in the diet. Less than 2g of these bad fats is ideal in a serving of food. Look for products with higher amounts of monounsaturated and polyunsaturated fat as these are healthier than trans and saturated fat. Also, watch for elevated sodium levels (i.e. suggested maximum Canadian daily value is 1500mg) as excessive salt in processed foods may increase the risk of developing high blood pressure. More positively, look for high amounts of fibre (more than 5 g) and vitamins and minerals. Also, do not forget to look at the serving size indicated on the nutritional facts panel. The serving size is dictated by Canadian regulations to ensure the amount is portion appropriate. You can use the serving size as a guideline as to what would be an appropriate amount of that type of food to eat.

d) Food Products to Consider

Champlain Valley – organic frozen fruits and vegetables available in a variety of options.

Crofters – a line of organic jams from natural fruits.
http://www.croftersorganic.com

Eden Organic – a line of a large variety of organic canned goods including beans and vegetables. http://www.edenfoods.com

Healthy Times – a natural baby and junior food line that includes the nutritional ideas discussed here
http://www.healthytimes.com

Just Juice – an all natural, not from concentrate juice line with no added sugar. Most of the line is certified organic. www.vervenaturals.com

Nature's Path – a line of cereals with quality complex carbohydrates. Look for those cereals with higher protein counts. www.naturespath.com

Nuts to You – various nut butters with no trans fat, hydrogenated oils or other undesirable additives.

Purely Bulk – a line of bulk natural foods in convenient plastic tubs. Offers some of the more natural sugars and whole grains. www.purelybulk.com

Spectrum Naturals – a line of quality organic oils, including organic olive oil. www.spectrumnaturals.com

e) Healthy Snacks to Look For

In Your Face Snacks – small bagged nuts and seeds at an affordable price, these great snack bags make eating nuts and seeds a portable, fun snack. www.inyourfacesnacks.com

Kettle Valley Organic Fruit Snacks – made with organic fruit and with no added sugar or preservatives this bar is a great way to pack fruits into your diet while on the run. www.kettlevalley.net

Real Organic Bars – dried organic fruit and/or vegetable bars available in a number of varieties including green, berry, tropical and blueberry flax. Being high in fibre and loaded with antioxidants these are a very healthy snack. www.realgreen.ca

Virta Organic Raw Sprout Bar – high in fibre, antioxidant rich vegetable or berry blends, and with sprouted grains and soy, this is the ultimate snack as it tastes good, is very portable and full of good ingredients. With a mix of complex carbs, plant products and soy protein this is a great snack when on the run. www.vervenaturals.com

f) Supplements

Herbal Select - a complete line of essential fatty acids including a unique vegetarian 369 formula. Pharmaceutical grade and free of mercury, PCBs and other contaminants. Oils provided by Canada's award winning fatty acid supplier, Bioriginal. www.herbalselect.com

NOW Foods – one of the best known natural supplement suppliers. They offer one of the widest varieties of quality supplements, each ensured to be of high quality and at an affordable price. Products offered continuously grow to represent the most current scientifically supported discoveries. Have a helpful website for supplement information. www.nowfoods.com

Nutrition Now – probiotic manufacturer with a scientifically supported blend of eight probiotic strains. They are known for quality and high dosage delivery. www.nutritionnow.com

Sequel Naturals - a line of supplements created with the most current technology and from a high quality specialized supply. Products include Vega, a vegan, organic meal replacement mixture with a clean ingredient list. www.sequelnaturals.com

References:

[1]Shade ED, Ulrich CM, Wener MH, Wood B, Yasui Y, Lacroix K, Potter JD, McTiernan A. Frequent intentional weight loss is associated with lower natural killer cell cytotoxicity in postmenopausal women: possible long-term immune effects. Journal of American Dietetic Association. 2004 Jun;104(6):903-12.

[2]Dr. Keith Garleib. Annual Meeting and Food Expo at the Institute of Food and Technologists, 2004.

[3]Willett WC, and Leibel RL. Dietary fat is not a major determinant of body fat. Am J Med 2002, Dec 113:47S-59S.

[4]Grocery Manufacturers of America Survey, 2003.

[5]Blackburn GL, Phillips JC and Morreale S. Physicians guide to popular low-carbohydrate weight loss diets. Cleve Clin J Med 2001, 68(9):761-773.

[6]McGinnis JM, Foege WH. Actual causes of death in the United States. JAMA. 1993 Nov 10;270(18):2207-12.

[7]National Health and Nutrition Examination Survey (NHANES), 2000.

[8]International Association for the Study of Obesity. 2003. http://www.iotf.org/

[9]Unknown. Check Up, 2004;15:23-2.

[10]Calle EE, Rodriguez C, Walker-Thurmond K, Thun MJ. Overweight, obesity, and mortality from cancer in a prospectively studied cohort of U.S. adults. N Engl J Med. 2003 Apr 24;348(17):1625-38.

[11]van Baak MA. Exercise training and substrate utilisation in obesity. Int J Obes Relat Metab Disord. 1999 Apr;23 Suppl 3:S11-7.

[12]Votruba SB, Horvitz MA, Schoeller DA. The role of exercise in the treatment of obesity. Nutrition. 2000 Mar;16(3):179-88.

[13]Ross R, Janssen I. Physical activity, total and regional obesity: dose-response considerations. Med Sci Sports Exerc. 2001 Jun;33(6 Suppl):S52-7.

[14]Jakicic JM, Marcus BH, Gallagher KI, Napolitano M, Lang W. Effect of exercise duration and intensity on weight loss in overweight, sedentary women: a randomized trial. JAMA. 2003 Sep 10;290(10):1323-30.

[15, 16]Hansen K, Shriver T, Schoeller D. The effects of exercise on the storage and oxidation of dietary fat. Sports Med 2005: 35(5):363-373.

[17]Unknown. Low-Carbohydrate Diets: Do they work? Mayo Clinic Women's HealthSource. October 2003.

[18]Bravata DM, Sanders L, Huang J, Krumholz HM, Olkin I, Gardner CD, Bravata DM. Efficacy and safety of low-carbohydrate diets: a systematic review. JAMA. 2003 Apr 9;289(14):1837-50.

[19]Time Magazine. 'The Low-carb Food Craze', May 3, 2004.

[20]Bravata DM, Sanders L, Huang J, Krumholz HM, Olkin I, Gardner CD, Bravata DM. Efficacy and safety of low-carbohydrate diets: a systematic review. JAMA. 2003 Apr 9;289(14):1837-50.

[21]Foster GD, Wyatt HR, Hill JO, McGuckin BG, Brill C, Mohammed BS, Szapary PO, Rader DJ, Edman JS, Klein S. A randomized trial of a low-carbohydrate diet for obesity. N Engl J Med. 2003 May 22;348(21):2082-90.

[22]Brehm BJ, Seeley RJ, Daniels SR, D'Alessio DA. A randomized trial comparing a very low-carbohydrate diet and a calorie-restricted low fat diet on body weight and

cardiovascular risk factors in healthy women. J Clin Endocrinol Metab. 2003 Apr;88(4):1617-23.

[23]Bravata DM, Sanders L, Huang J, Krumholz HM, Olkin I, Gardner CD, Bravata DM. Efficacy and safety of low-carbohydrate diets: a systematic review. JAMA. 2003 Apr 9;289(14):1837-50.

[24]Samuel P. Fibres Effect on Childhood Obesity. *Presented at* Experimental Biology Conference, 2003; Apr 11-15.

[25]Saris, WH. Sugars, energy metabolism, and body weight control. Am J Clin Nutr. 2003 Oct;78(4):850S-857S.

[26]Blundell JE, and Stubbs RJ. High and low-carbohydrate and fat intakes: limits imposed by appetite and palatability and their implications for energy balance. Eur J Clin Nutr,1999 Apr;53:S148-65.

[27]National Mental Health Association, USA, 1996.

[28]Volek JS, and Westman EC. Very low-carbohydrate weight loss diets revisited. Cleve Clin J Med. 2002 Nov;69(11):849-58.

[29]Ludwig, DS. Dietary glycemic index and the regulation of body weight. Lipids. 2003;38(2):117-21.

[30]Steffansson. *The Effects of an Exclusive Long-Continued Meat Diet.* Journal of American Medical Association.

[31]Keys A, Aravanis C, Blackburn HW, Van Buchem FSP, Buzina R, Djordjevic BS, Dontas AS, Fidanza F, Karvonen MJ, Kimura N, Lekos D, Monti M, Puddu V, Taylor HL. Epidemiologic studies related to coronary heart disease: characteristics of men aged 40-59 in seven countries. Acta Med Scand 1967 (Suppl to vol. 460) 1-392.

[32]Keys A. Seven countries: a multivariate analysis of death and coronary heart disease. London: Harvard University Press, 1980.

[33]Atkins, Robert C. Atkins for Life. 2003. St. Martin's Press, New York, NY.

[34]Sanchez A, Reeser JL, Lau HS, Yahiku PY, Willard RE, McMillan PJ, Cho SY, Magie AR, Register UD. Role of sugars in human neutrophilic phagocytosis Am J Clin Nutr Nov, 1973;261:1180-84.

[35]Nieman DC, Fagoaga OR, Butterworth DE, Warren BJ, Utter A, Davis JM, Henson DA, Nehlsen –Cannarella SL. Carbohydrate supplementation affects blood granulocyte and monocyte trafficking but not function after 2.5 h of running. Am J Clin Nutr. 1997 Jul;66(1):153-9.

[36]Scott AR, Attenborough Y, Peacock I, Fletcher E, Jeffcoate WJ, Tattersall RB. Comparison of high fibre diets, basal insulin supplements, and flexible insulin treatment for non-insulin dependent (type II) diabetics poorly controlled with sulphonylureas. BMJ. 1988 Sep 17;297(6650):707-10.

[37]Mady MA, Kossoff EH, McGregor AL, Wheless JW, Pyzik PL, Freeman JM. The ketogenic diet: adolescents can do it, too. Epilepsia. 2003 Jun;44(6):847-51.

[38]Liu S, Willett WC, Manson JE, Hu FB, Rosner B, Colditz G. Relation between changes in intakes of dietary fiber and grain products and changes in weight and development of obesity among middle-aged women. Am J Clin Nutr. 2003;78(5):920-927.

[39]Cheuvront SN. The Zone Diet phenomenon: a closer look at the science behind the claims. J Am Coll Nutr. 2003 Feb;22(1):9-17.

[40]Vermunt, SH, et al. Effects of sugar intake on body weight: a review. Obes Rev. 2003 May; 4(2):91-9.

[41]Foster GD, Wyatt HR, Hill JO, McGuckin BG, Brill C, Mohammed BS, Szapary PO, Rader DJ, Edman JS, Klein S. A randomized trial of a low-carbohydrate diet for

obesity. N Engl J Med. 2003 May 22;348(21):2082-90.

[42]Brehm BJ, Seeley RJ, Daniels SR, D'Alessio DA. A randomized trial comparing a very low-carbohydrate diet and a calorie-restricted low fat diet on body weight and cardiovascular risk factors in healthy women. J Clin Endocrinol Metab. 2003 Apr;88(4):1617-23.

[43]Anderson JW, Konz EC, Jenkins DJ. Health advantages and disadvantages of weight-reducing diets: a computer analysis and critical review. J Am Coll Nutr. 2000 Oct;19(5):578-90.

[44]Sommariva D, Scotti L, Fasoli A. Low-fat diet versus low-carbohydrate diet in the treatment of type IV hyperlipoproteinaemia. Atherosclerosis. 1978 Jan;29(1):43-51.

[45]Mathieson RA, Walberg JL, Gwazdauskas FC, Hinkle DE, Gregg JM. The effect of varying carbohydrate content of a very-low-caloric diet on resting metabolic rate and thyroid hormones. Metabolism. 1986 May;35(5):394-8.

[46]Ipsos Reid. January 2004.

[47]Ipsos Reid January 2004.

[48]Thompson HJ, Heimendinger J, Haegele A, Sedlacek SM, Gillette C, O'Neill C, Wolfe P, Conry C. Effect of increased vegetable and fruit consumption on markers of oxidative cellular damage. Carcinogenesis. 1999 Dec;20(12):2261-6.

[49]Jenkins DJ, Kendall CW, Marchie A, Jenkins AL, Connelly PW, Jones PJ, Vuksan V. The Garden of Eden--plant based diets, the genetic drive to conserve cholesterol and its implications for heart disease in the 21st century. Comp Biochem Physiol A Mol Integr Physiol. 2003 Sep;136(1):141-51.

[50]Joseph JA, Shukitt-Hale B, Denisova NA, Bielinski D, Martin A, McEwen JJ, Bickford PC. Reversals of age-related declines in neuronal signal transduction, cognitive, and motor behavioral deficits with blueberry, spinach, or strawberry dietary supplementation. J Neurosci. 1999 Sep 15;19(18):8114-21.

[51]Philpott M, Ferguson LR. Immunonutrition and cancer. Mutat Res. 2004 Jul 13;551(1-2):29-42.

[52]Suthar AC, Banavalikar MM, Biyani MK. Pharmacological activities of Genistein, an isoflavone from soy (Glycine max): part I--anti-cancer activity. Indian J Exp Biol. 2001 Jun;39(6):511-9.

[53]Arliss RM, Biermann CA. Do soy isoflavones lower cholesterol, inhibit atherosclerosis, and play a role in cancer prevention? Holist Nurs Pract. 2002 Oct;16(5):40-8.

[54]Chen J, Stavro PM, Thompson LU. Dietary flaxseed inhibits human breast cancer growth and metastasis and downregulates expression of insulin-like growth factor and epidermal growth factor receptor. Nutr Cancer. 2002;43(2):187-92.

[55]Haggans CJ, Hutchins AM, Olson BA, Thomas W, Martini MC, Slavin JL. Effect of flaxseed consumption on urinary estrogen metabolites in postmenopausal women. Nutr Cancer. 1999;33(2):188-95.

[56]Kerstetter JE, O'Brien KO, Insogna KL. Dietary protein, calcium metabolism, and skeletal homeostasis revisited. Am J Clin Nutr. 2003 Sep;78(3 Suppl):584S-592S.

[57]McGill NW. Gout and other crystal-associated arthropathies. Baillieres Best Pract Res Clin Rheumatol. 2000 Sep;14(3):445-60.

[58]Walker JD, Bending JJ, Dodds RA, Mattock MB, Murrells TJ, Keen H, Viberti GC Restriction of dietary protein and progression of renal failure in diabetic nephropathy. Lancet. 1989 Dec 16;2(8677):1411-5.

[59]Barzel US, Massey LK. Excess dietary protein can adversely affect bone. J Nutr. 1998 Jun;128(6):1051-3.

[60]Sachiko T. St. Jeor, Barbara V. Howard, T. Elaine Prewitt, Vicki Bovee, Terry Bazzarre, and Robert H. Eckel. Dietary Protein and Weight Reduction: A Statement for Healthcare Professionals from the Nutrition Committee of the Council on Nutrition, Physical Activity, and Metabolism of the American Heart Association. Circulation 2001 104: 1869 - 1874.

[61]Singh PN, Sabate J, Fraser GE. Does low meat consumption increase life expectancy in humans? Am J Clin Nutr. 2003 Sep;78(3 Suppl):526S-532S

[62]Barzel US, Massey LK. Excess dietary protein can adversely affect bone. J Nutr. 1998 Jun;128(6):1051-3.

[63]Dawson-Hughes B, Harris SS, Rasmussen H, Song L, Dallal GE. Effect of dietary protein supplements on calcium excretion in healthy older men and women. J Clin Endocrinol Metab. 2004 Mar;89(3):1169-73.

[64]Heaney RP. Excess dietary protein may not adversely affect bone. J Nutr. 1998 Jun;128(6):1054-7.

[65]Kerstetter JE, O'Brien KO, Insogna KL. Dietary protein, calcium metabolism, and skeletal homeostasis revisited. Am J Clin Nutr. 2003 Sep;78(3 Suppl):584S-592S.

[66]Clifton PM, Noakes M, Keogh J, Foster P. Effect of an energy reduced high protein red meat diet on weight loss and metabolic parameters in obese women. Asia Pac J Clin Nutr. 2003;12 Suppl:S10.

[67]Bowen J, Noakes M, Clifton P. High dairy-protein versus high mixed-protein energy restricted diets - the effect on bone turnover and calcium excretion in overweight adults. Asia Pac J Clin Nutr. 2003;12 Suppl:S52.

[68]Unknown. Diet and Bones. Am J Clin Nutr. 1978;31:167-168.

[69]Tylavsky FA, Holliday K, Danish R, Womack C, Norwood J, Carbone L. Fruit and vegetable intakes are an independent predictor of bone size in early pubertal children. Am J Clin Nutr. 2004 Feb;79(2):311-7.

[70]Claire P McGartland, Paula J Robson, Liam J Murray, Gordon W Cran, Maurice J Savage, David C Watkins, Madeleine M Rooney and Colin A Boreham. American Journal of Clinical Nutrition, 80(4);1019-1023.

[71]Larosa JC. Effects of high-protein, low-carbohydrate dieting on plasma lipoproteins and body weight. J Am Diet Assoc. 1980 Sep;77(3):264-70.

[72]Gordon T, et al. Diabetes, blood lipids, and the role of obesity in coronary heart disease risk for women. The Framingham study. Ann Intern Med. 1977 Oct;87(4):393-7.

[73]Stone NJ. Diet, lipids, and coronary heart disease. Endocrinol Metab Clin North Am. 1990 Jun;19(2):321-44.

[74]Hu FB, Rimm EB, Stampfer MJ, Ascherio A, Spiegelman D, Willett WC. Prospective study of major dietary patterns and risk of coronary heart disease in men. Am J Clin Nutr. 2000 Oct;72(4):912-21.

[75]Jenkins DJ, Kendall CW, Marchie A, Jenkins AL, Connelly PW, Jones PJ, Vuksan V. The Garden of Eden--plant based diets, the genetic drive to conserve cholesterol and its implications for heart disease in the 21st century. Comp Biochem Physiol A Mol Integr Physiol. 2003 Sep;136(1):141-51.

[76]Roche HM. Dietary carbohydrates and triacylglycerol metabolism. Proc Nutr Soc. Feb 1999, 58(1):201-7.

[77]Prentice AM, Jebb SA. Fast foods, energy density and obesity: a possible mechanistic link.
Obes Rev. 2003 Nov;4(4):187-94.

[78]Steyn NP, Mann J, Bennett PH, Temple N, Zimmet P, Tuomilehto J, Lindstrom J, Louheranta A. Diet, nutrition and the prevention of type 2 diabetes. Public Health

Nutr. 2004 Feb;7(1A):147-65.
[79]Steyn NP, Mann J, Bennett PH, Temple N, Zimmet P, Tuomilehto J, Lindstrom J, Louheranta A. Diet, nutrition and the prevention of type 2 diabetes. Public Health Nutr. 2004 Feb;7(1A):147-65.
[80]Kelley DE. Sugars and starch in the nutritional management of diabetes mellitus. Am J Clin Nutr. 2003 Oct;78(4):858S-864S.
[81]Bertone ER, Rosner BA, Hunter DJ, Stampfer MJ, Speizer FE, Colditz GA, Willett WC, Hankinson SE. Dietary fat intake and ovarian cancer in a cohort of US women. Am J Epidemiol. 2002 Jul 1;156(1):22-31.
[82]Moyad MA. Selenium and vitamin E supplements for prostate cancer: evidence or embellishment? Urology. 2002 Apr;59(4 Suppl 1):9-19.
[83]Bruce WR, Wolever TM, Giacca A. Mechanisms linking diet and colorectal cancer: the possible role of insulin resistance. Nutr Cancer. 2000;37(1):19-26.
[84]Hawley JA, Dennis SC, Noakes TD. Oxidation of carbohydrate ingested during prolonged endurance exercise. Sports Med. 1992 Jul;14(1):27-42.
[85]Barnard ND, and Lanou, AJ. Analysis of Health Problems Associated with High-Protein, High-Fat, Carbohydrate-Restricted Diets Reported via an Online Registry. Physicians Committee for Responsible Medicine. http://www.pcrm.org/news/registry_report.html. Updated May 25, 2004.
[86]Unknown. Low-carbs cause mood 'lows'. Nutraingredients, March 2, 2004.
[87]Bilsborough SA, Crowe TC. Low-carbohydrate diets: what are the potential short- and long-term health implications? Asia Pac J Clin Nutr. 2003;12(4):396-404.
[88]Wolever, TM. Carbohydrate and the regulation of blood glucose and metabolism. Nutr Rev. 2003;61:S40-8.
[89]Brand-Miller J, Hayne S, Petocz P, Colagiuri S. Low-glycemic index diets in the management of diabetes: a meta-analysis of randomized controlled trials. Diabetes Care, Aug;26(8):2261-7.
[90]Pelkman CL. Effects of the glycemic index of foods on serum concentrations on high-density lipoprotein cholesterol and triglycerides. Curr Atheroscler Rep. 2001. Nov 3(6):456-61.
[91]Dietary Reference Intakes. The National Academies, 1998.
[92]Bailey LB. Folate, methyl-related nutrients, alcohol, and the MTHFR 677C-->T polymorphism affect cancer risk: intake recommendations. J Nutr. 2003 Nov;133 (11 Suppl 1):3748S-3753S.
[93]CDC, National Center for Health Statistics. Colorectal Cancer Death Rates Among Men and Women, by Race and Ethnicity, United States, 1990—2000.
[94]Gardner, D. High protein diet may be bad for women trying to conceive. European Society of Human Reproduction and Embryology Conference. Abstract 0-076. June 28,2004.
[95]Taylor PD, Khan IY, Hanson MA, Poston L. Impaired EDHF-mediated vasodilatation in adult offspring of rats exposed to a fat-rich diet in pregnancy. J Physiol. 2004 Aug 1;558(Pt 3):943-51. Epub 2004 Jun 11.
[96]Vegetarians go low-carb. Guelph Mercury. May 12, 2004; B1.
[97]Ikeda K, Harada Y and Okamura K. Preference For Sweetness May Decrease After Exercise In Rats. Experimental Biology 2004 Conference. Abstract # 2662.
[98]Brown RC. Nutrition for optimal performance during exercise: carbohydrate and fat. Curr Sports Med Rep. 2002 Aug;1(4):222-9.
[99]Burke LM, Kiens B, Ivy JL. Carbohydrates and fat for training and recovery. J Sports Sci. 2004 Jan;22(1):15-30.

100Johnson NA, Stannard SR, Thompson MW. Muscle triglyceride and glycogen in endurance exercise: implications for performance. Sports Med. 2004;34(3):151-64.
101Burke LM, Kiens B, Ivy JL. Carbohydrates and fat for training and recovery. J Sports Sci. 2004 Jan;22(1):15-30.
102Hawley JA, Dennis SC, Noakes TD. Oxidation of carbohydrate ingested during prolonged endurance exercise. Sports Med. 1992 Jul;14(1):27-42
103Romieu1 S, Lazcano-Ponce1 E, Sanchez-Zamorano1 LM, Willett W and Hernandez-Avila1 M. Carbohydrates and the Risk of Breast Cancer among Mexican Women. Journal of Cancer Epidemiology Biomarkers in Prevention. 2004: 13, 1283-1289.
104National Health and Nutrition Examination Survey (NHANES), 2000.
105International Association for the Study of Obesity. 2003. http://www.iotf.org/
106 Lacey JV Jr, Swanson CA, Brinton LA, Altekruse SF, Barnes WA, Gravitt PE, Greenberg MD, Hadjimichael OC, McGowan L, Mortel R, Schwartz PE, Kurman RJ, Hildesheim A. Obesity as a potential risk factor for adenocarcinomas and squamous cell carcinomas of the uterine cervix. Cancer. 2003 Aug 15;98(4):814-21.
107Astrup A, Gotzsche PC, van de Werken K, Ranneries C, Toubro S, Raben A, Buemann B. Meta-analysis of resting metabolic rate in formerly obese subjects. Am J Clin Nutr. 1999 Jun;69(6):1117-22.
108Kral T, Roe L, and Rolls B.The Combined Effects of Energy Density and Portion Size on Food and Energy Intake in Women. North American Association for the Study of Obesity Meeting Oct 13, 2003.
109Dallman MF, Pecoraro N, Akana SF, la Fleur SE, Gomez F, Houshyar H, Bell ME, Bhatnagar S, Laugero KD, and Manalo S. Chronic stress and obesity: A new view of "comfort food". PNAS 2003 100: 11696-11701.
110Dallman MF, Pecoraro N, Akana SF, la Fleur SE, Gomez F, Houshyar H, Bell ME, Bhatnagar S, Laugero KD, and Manalo S. Chronic stress and obesity: A new view of "comfort food". PNAS 2003 100: 11696-11701.
111Lambert, C. The Way We Eat Now: Ancient bodies collide with modern technology to produce a flabby, disease-ridden populace. Harvard Magazine. 2004: 106(5), 50.
112Sanders, T. High-versus low-fat diets in human diseases. Curr Opin Clin Nutr Metab Care. 2003;6(2):151-5.
113Mensink RPM, Katan MB. Effect of dietary trans fatty acids on high-density and low-density lipoprotein cholesterol levels in healthy subjects. N Engl J Med 1990; 323:439-45.
114Willett WC, Ascherio A. Trans fatty acids: Are the effects only marginal? Am J Public Health 1994; 84:722-724
115Expert Panel on Trans Fatty Acids and Coronary Heart Disease. Trans fatty acids and coronary heart disease risk. Am J Clin Nutr 1995; 62:655S-708S.
116Wolfram, G. Dietary fatty acids and coronary heart disease. Eur J Med Res. 2003 Aug 20;8(8):321-4.
117Watkins BA, Li Y, Seifert MF. Nutraceutical fatty acids as biochemical and molecular modulators of skeletal. J Am Coll Nutr. 2001 Oct;20(5 Suppl):410S-416S; discussion 417S-420S.
118Ziboh VA, Miller CC, Cho Y. Significance of lipoxygenase-derived monohydroxy fatty acids in cutaneous biology. Prostaglandins Other Lipid Mediat. 2000 Nov;63 (1-2):3-13.
119Li D. Omega-3 fatty acids and non-communicable diseases. Chin Med J. 2003 Mar;116(3):453-8.
120J. A. Menendez, L. Vellon, R. Colomer, and R. Lupu. Oleic acid, the main

monounsaturated fatty acid of olive oil, suppresses Her-2/neu (erbB-2) expression and synergistically enhances the growth inhibitory effects of trastuzumab (HerceptinTM) in breast cancer cells with Her-2/neu oncogene amplification. Annuals of Oncology, Advance Access published on January 10, 2005.
[121]Lichtenstein AH, Kennedy E, Barrier P, Danford D, Ernst ND, Grundy SM, Leveille GA, Van Horn L, Williams CL, Booth SL. Dietary fat consumption and health. Nutr Rev. 1998 May;56(5 Pt 2):S3-19; discussion S19-28.
[122]Steinhart H, Rickert R, Winkler K. Trans fatty acids (TFA): analysis, occurrence, intake and clinical relevance. Eur J Med Res. 2003 Aug 20;8(8):358-62.
[123]Naruszewicz M, Daniewski M, Nowicka G, Kozlowska-Wojciechowska M. Trans-unsaturated fatty acids and acrylamide in food as potential atherosclerosis progression factors. Based on own studies. Acta Microbiol Pol. 2003;52 Suppl:75-81.
[124]Mojska, H. Influence of trans fatty acids on infant and fetus development. Acta Microbiol Pol. 2003;52 Suppl:67-74.
[125]Nordoy A. Statins and omega-3 fatty acids in the treatment of dyslipidemia and coronary heart disease. Minerva Med. 2002 Oct;93(5):357-63.
[126]No Author Listed. Dietary supplementation with n-3 polyunsaturated fatty acids and vitamin E after myocardial infarction: results of the GISSI-Prevenzione trial. Lancet. 1999 Aug 7;354(9177):447-55.
[127]American Heart Association, 2000.
[128]Skoldstam L, Hagfors L, Johansson G. An experimental study of a Mediterranean diet intervention for patients with rheumatoid arthritis. Ann Rheum Dis. 2003 Mar;62(3):208-14.
[129]Belch JJ, Ansell D, Madhok R, O'Dowd A, and Sturrock RD. Effects of altering dietary essential fatty acids on requirements for non-steroidal anti-inflammatory drugs in patients with rheumatoid arthritis: a double blind placebo controlled study. Ann Rheum Dis 1988; 47: 96-104.
[130]Remans PH, Sont JK, Wagenaar LW, Wouters-Wesseling W, Zuijderduin WM, Jongma A, Breedveld FC, Van Laar JM. Nutrient supplementation with polyunsaturated fatty acids and micronutrients in rheumatoid arthritis: clinical and biochemical effects. Eur J Clin Nutr. 2004 Jun;58(6):839-45.
[131]al-Shabanah OA. Effect of evening primrose oil on gastric ulceration and secretion induced by various ulcerogenic and necrotizing agents in rats. Food Chem Toxicol. 1997 Aug;35(8):769-75.
[132]Young GS, Maharaj NJ, Conquer JA. Blood phospholipid fatty acid analysis of adults with and without attention deficit/hyperactivity disorder. Lipids. 2004 Feb;39(2):117-23.
[133]Ross BM, McKenzie I, Glen I, Bennett CP. Increased levels of ethane, a non-invasive marker of n-3 fatty acid oxidation, in breath of children with attention deficit hyperactivity disorder. Nutr Neurosci. 2003 Oct;6(5):277-81.
[134]Hardman, W.E. Omega-3 fatty acids to Augment Cancer Therapy. J. Nutr. 2002; 132:3508S-3512S.
[135]Das UN. Gamma-linolenic acid, arachidonic acid, and eicosapentaenoic acid as potential anticancer drugs. Nutrition. 1990 Nov-Dec;6(6):429-34.
[136]Hutchins A, Martin M, Olson B, Thomas W, Slavin J. Flaxseed influences urinary lignan excretion in a dose-dependent manner in postmenopausal women. Cancer, Epidemiology, Biomarkers and Prevention, 2000;9:1113-1118.
[137]Flaxseed Shows Promise Against Breast Cancer. American Institute for Cancer

Research Newsletter, 1998; 59.

[138]Joshi S, Rao S, Golwilkar A, Patwardhan M, Bhonde R. Fish oil supplementation of rats during pregnancy reduces adult disease risks in their offspring. J Nutr. 2003 Oct;133(10):3170-4.

[139]Togni V, Ota CC, Folador A, Junior OT, Aikawa J, Yamazaki RK, Freitas FA, Longo R, Martins EF, Calder PC, Curi R, Fernandes LC. Cancer cachexia and tumor growth reduction in Walker 256 tumor-bearing rats supplemented with N-3 polyunsaturated fatty acids for one generation.
Nutr Cancer. 2003;46(1):52-8.

[140]Malcolm CA, McCulloch DL, Montgomery C, Shepherd A, Weaver LT. Maternal docosahexaenoic acid supplementation during pregnancy and visual evoked potential development in term infants: a double blind, prospective, randomized trial. Arch Dis Child Fetal Neonatal Ed. 2003 Sep;88(5):F383-90.

[141]Duttaroy AK. Fetal growth and development: roles of fatty acid transport proteins and nuclear transcription factors in human placenta. Indian J Exp Biol. 2004 Aug;42(8):747-57.

[142]Crawford MA, Golfetto I, Ghebremeskel K, Min Y, Moodley T, Poston L, Phylactos A, Cunnane S, Schmidt W. The potential role for arachidonic and docosahexaenoic acids in protection against some central nervous system injuries in preterm infants. Lipids. 2003 Apr;38(4):303-15

[143]Gaullier JM, Halse J, Hoye K, Kristiansen K, Fagertun H, Vik H, Gudmundsen O. Conjugated linoleic acid supplementation for 1 y reduces body fat mass in healthy overweight humans. Am J Clin Nutr. 2004 Jun;79(6):1118-25.

[144]Ntambi JM, Choi Y, Park Y, Peters JM, Pariza MW. Effects of conjugated linoleic acid (CLA) on immune responses, body composition and stearoyl-CoA desaturase. Can J Appl Physiol. 2002 Dec;27(6):617-28.

[145]DeLany JP, West DB. Changes in body composition with conjugated linoleic acid. J Am Coll Nutr. 2000 Aug;19(4):487S-493S

[146]Rahman SM, Wang Y, Yotsumoto H, Cha J, Han S, Inoue S, Yanagita T. Effects of conjugated linoleic acid on serum leptin concentration, body-fat accumulation, and beta-oxidation of fatty acid in OLETF rats. Nutrition. 2001 May;17(5):385-90

[147]Belury MA, Mahon A, Banni S. The conjugated linoleic acid (CLA) isomer, t10c12-CLA, is inversely associated with changes in body weight and serum leptin in subjects with type 2 diabetes mellitus. J Nutr. 2003 Jan;133(1):257S-260S.

[148]Ntambi JM, Choi Y, Park Y, Peters JM, Pariza MW. Effects of conjugated linoleic acid (CLA) on immune responses, body composition and stearoyl-CoA desaturase. Can J Appl Physiol. 2002 Dec;27(6):617-28.

[149]O'Hagan S, Menzel A. A subchronic 90-day oral rat toxicity study and in vitro genotoxicity studies with a conjugated linoleic acid product. Food Chem Toxicol. 2003 Dec;41(12):1749-60.

[150]Scimeca JA. Toxicological evaluation of dietary conjugated linoleic acid in male Fischer 344 rats.
Food Chem Toxicol. 1998 May;36(5):391-5.

[151]Riserus U, Basu S, Jovinge S, Fredrikson GN, Arnlov J, Vessby B. Supplementation with conjugated linoleic acid causes isomer-dependent oxidative stress and elevated C-reactive protein: a potential link to fatty acid-induced insulin resistance. Circulation. 2002 Oct 8;106(15):1925-9.

[152]Riserus U, Arner P, Brismar K, Vessby B. Treatment with dietary trans10cis12 conjugated linoleic acid causes isomer-specific insulin resistance in obese men with

the metabolic syndrome. Diabetes Care. 2002 Sep;25(9):1516-21.
[153]Colagiuri S, Brand Miller J. The 'carnivore connection'--evolutionary aspects of insulin resistance. Eur J Clin Nutr. 2002 Mar;56 Suppl 1:S30-5.
[154]Franz MJ. Protein and diabetes: much advice, little research. Curr Diab Rep. 2002 Oct;2(5):457-64
[155]Times Magazine. The Low-Carb Food Craze. May 3, 2004.
[156]Unknown. The Thin Science of Fad Diets. Wired Magazine December 2003.
[157]Barzi F, Woodward M, Marfisi RM, Tavazzi L, Valagussa F, Marchioli R; GISSI-Prevenzione Investigators. Mediterranean diet and all-causes mortality after myocardial infarction: results from the GISSI-Prevenzione trial. Eur J Clin Nutr. 2003 Apr;57(4):604-11.
[158]Zemel MB, et al. Dietary Calcium and Dairy Products Accelerate Weight and Fat Loss During Energy Restriction in Obese Adults. Obesity Research. 2004; 12(4): 582-590.
[159]Jenkins D, Kendall C, Marchie A, Faulkner D, Wong J, de Souza R, Emam A, Parker T, Vidgen E, Trautwein E, Lapsley K, Josse R, Leiter L, Singer W, and Connelly P. Direct comparison of a dietary portfolio of cholesterol-lowering foods with a statin in hypercholesterolemic participants. Am J Clin Nutr 2005 81: 380-387.
[160]Tucker KL, Hannan MT, Kiel DP. The acid-base hypothesis: diet and bone in the Framingham Osteoporosis Study. Eur J Nutr. 2001 Oct;40(5):231-7.
[161]Pereira MA. Breakfast and Diabetes. Presented at the American Heart Association's 43rd Annual Conference on Cardiovascular Disease Epidemiology and Prevention, March 5-8, 2003, Miami.
[162]Holt SH, Miller JC, Petocz P, Farmakalidis E. A satiety index of common foods. Eur J Clin Nutr. 1995 Sep;49(9):675-90.
[163]Kral, A. Calorie density and consumption. Presented at the Annual North American Assoc for the Study of Obesity in Florida, Oct 11-15, 2003.
[164]Dallman MF, Pecoraro N, Akana SF, La Fleur SE, Gomez F, Houshyar H, Bell ME, Bhatnagar S, Laugero KD, Manalo S. Chronic stress and obesity: a new view of "comfort food". Proc Natl Acad Sci U S A. 2003 Sep 30;100(20):11696-701.
[165]Opinion Dynmanics Corporation, August 2004.
[166]Wang YW, Jones PJ. Conjugated linoleic acid and obesity control: efficacy and mechanisms. Int J Obes Relat Metab Disord. 2004 Aug;28(8):941-55.
[167]Jacqmain M, Doucet E, Despres JP, Bouchard C, Tremblay A. Calcium intake, body composition, and lipoprotein-lipid concentrations in adults. Am J Clin Nutr. 2003 Jun;77(6):1448-52.
[168]Ishitani K, Itakura E, Goto S, Esashi T. Calcium absorption from the ingestion of coral-derived calcium by humans. J Nutr Sci Vitaminol 1999, 45:509-1.
[169]Kenny AM, Prestwood KM, Biskup B, Robbins B, Zayas E, Kleppinger A, Burleson JA, Raisz LG Comparison of the effects of calcium loading with calcium citrate or calcium carbonate on bone turnover in postmenopausal women. Osteoporos Int. 2004 Apr;15(4):290-4. Epub 2004 Jan 13.
[170]Continuing Survey of Food Intakes by Individuals (1994-1996). US Department of Agriculture. 1998.
[171]Reid, G. The Scientific Basis for Probiotic Strains of Lactobacillus. Applied Environ Microbiol, 1999; 9 (65): 3763-3766.
[172]Timmerman HM, Koning CJ, Mulder L, Rombouts FM, Beynen AC. Monostrain, multistrain and multispecies probiotics – a comparison of functionality and efficacy. Int J Food Microbiol. 2004; 96(3):219-33.